AF553038

Cataract Surgery in Dogs

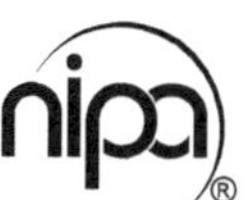

NIPA® GENX ELECTRONIC RESOURCES & SOLUTIONS P. LTD.
New Delhi-110 034

About the Author

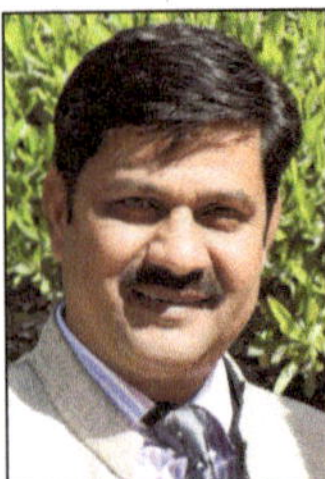

Dr. Suresh Kumar Jhirwal, Senior Assistant Professor, Department of Veterinary Surgery and Radiology is serving at College of Veterinary and Animal Science, Bikaner, Rajasthan University of Veterinary and Animal Sciences, Bikaner, since July 2014 after completing his successful tenure of 13 years and 7 months in the Department of Animal Husbandry, Government of Rajasthan.

After joining the University as an Assistant Professor he proved his work excellence as a Veterinary surgeon by contributing in new techniques i.e. Cataract surgery in dogs by Phacoemulsification and IOL implant using an operating microscope. He became the first Veterinary Surgeon of Rajasthan state to perform successful cataract surgery by phacoemulsification method in dogs. His work was recognised by the Rajasthan University of Veterinary and Animal Sciences, Bikaner, District administration, Bikaner, Government of Rajasthan, and many other organizations by felicitating him on various occasions.

In due course, he strengthened his skill and presented his work of ophthalmology on different platforms, and disseminated the knowledge. He won three consecutive GOLD MEDALs for best papers in the field of veterinary ophthalmology at the Annual congress of the Indian Society for Veterinary Surgery from 2017-2019.

He has guided 14 students in their masters' research out of which 11 conducted their research in the field of ophthalmology. He has 92 scientific publications to his credit and attended many conferences/symposiums/workshops of National and International repute. He is a member of six Scientific National and International organizations.

He is a popular invited expert to deliver offline delete or online technical lectures/ webinars on different topics for veterinary ophthalmology. He is committed to develop the diverse specialities of veterinary ophthalmology in a long way.

Cataract Surgery in Dogs

S.K. Jhirwal
Senior Assistant Professor,
Department of Veterinary Surgery and Radiology
College of Veterinary and Animal Science
Rajasthan University of Veterinary and Animal Sciences
Bikaner, Rajasthan

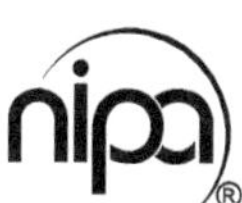

NIPA® GENX ELECTRONIC RESOURCES & SOLUTIONS P. LTD.
New Delhi-110 034

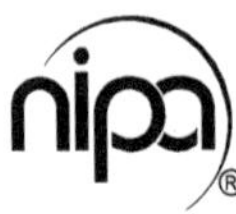

NIPA® GENX ELECTRONIC
RESOURCES & SOLUTIONS P. LTD.

101,103, Vikas Surya Plaza, CU Block
L.S.C.Market, Pitam Pura, New Delhi-110 034
Ph : +91 11 27341616, 27341717, 27341718
E-mail:newindiapublishingagency@gmail.com
www: www.nipabooks.com
For customer assistance, please contact
Phone: + 91-11-27 34 17 17
Fax: + 91-11-27 34 16 16
E-Mail: feedbacks@nipabooks.com

ISBN: 978-81-19002-64-1

Composed and Designed by NIPA®.

Acknowledgments

Writing a book is a collaborative effort and I would like to take this opportunity to thank all the people who have advised and encouraged me in this project.

At the outset, I bow my head to pay gratitude to my mentor a renowned scientist and worthy Professor T.K.Gahlot whose continuous motivation inspired me to learn the skills of veterinary ophthalmology which I never thought I would go. His keen interest in veterinary ophthalmology and zeal to procure required resources helped me to focus on the treatment, teaching, and research aspect of veterinary ophthalmology.

I also owe my heartfelt thanks to Dr. Sonia Gahlot, a human ophthalmologist; Dr. D.B.Patil, Professor, Veterinary Surgery, Kamdhenu University and Dr. Shasikant Mahajan, Professor, Veterinary Surgery, GADVASU are the persons who helped me to standardize the cataract surgery at CVAS, Bikaner. Their wholehearted support is acknowledged with much gratitude.

My special thanks goes to Dr. P. Bishnoi, Professor and Head, Veterinary Surgery and Radiology, CVAS, Bikaner for his unconditional support at the department.

Finally, I thank to my students who gave me the opportunity to strengthen my skills and academia in the field of veterinary ophthalmology while guiding them in their Master and Doctoral research projects.

Preface

Undoubtedly, Veterinary Ophthalmology developed with a slower pace in India because of lack of skilled personnels, inadequate instruments required for ophthalmic surgery of small and large animals and less number of availability of clinical cases. Gradually, owing to more awareness by pet and livestock owners they in turn had greater expectations from Veterinary Surgeons for application of advanced diagnostic and surgical procedures to treat the diverse ophthalmic affections. This was perhaps a triggering impetus to learn the modern veterinary ophthalmology and I got inspired to learn and develop this speciality in Clinic of my college.

Eventually, turning point came through the then Professor and Head, Dr T.K.Gahlot who succeeded to bring a well-funded project, i.e. Diagnostic Imaging and Management of Surgical Conditions of Animals (DIMSCA) from Indian Council of Agricultural Research (ICAR) through a visionary Deputy Director General- Prof. K.M.L.Pathak. Provisions were made to buy operating microscope, phacoemulsification and electroretinography instruments in addition to the basic ophthalmic surgery instruments. First exclusive small animal ophthalmic surgery operation theatre was established to standardize the diagnosis of diverse ophthalmic affections and cataract surgery in dogs. Prof. T.K. Gahlot further strengthened this speciality by procuring more ophthalmic instruments through Maharaja Ganga Singh Trust.

Ophthalmic surgery in small animals was done on clinical cases and became a part of clinical research at masters and doctorate level too. Cataract surgery in dogs was thus standardized with or without IOL employing either ECCE or phacoemulsification technique. An experienced team of medical and veterinary ophthalmologists also helped us from time to time while learning it.

The success story of operated cataract cases helped me to build up confidence and I not only continued doing cataract surgery in dogs but trained many vets and delivered several lectures through continuing education programmes organized by many veterinary colleges pan India. I am sure that the contents of this book would be a great help to those who are learning and practicing cataract surgery in pet animals.

Author

Contents

1

Introduction

Cataract is a common cause of visual impairment and blindness in dogs and has a wide variety of aetiologies, as well as the disabling effect on the animal. Cataracts present important welfare considerations for the owner. Visual impairment in dogs may lead to increased nervousness, aggression and reluctance to exercise, all of which may adversely affect the owner-pet relationship (1). The only effective mean of treatment for cataract is surgical extraction of diseased lens (2).

Although vision is one of the important faculties for any living individual, dogs have very well developed olfactory lobe and have great sense of smell. They can move about easily in limited area familiar to them even with impaired vision. Cataract surgery was therefore not a common procedure in animals for many years. Quite often however, when these dogs are exposed to unfamiliar surroundings or even otherwise sometimes, these affected dogs may stumble.

In recent years, many dog owners have shown keen interest in cataract surgery for their pets because cataract affects the vision of the dog and thus the utility. Cataract also affects the cosmetic look of the dog; some dogs may keep on banging and get injured. Due to deficit in the visual faculty, dogs affected with cataract frequently show anxiety and aggression as a defensive behaviour. To overcome this, cataract surgery is an indispensable remedy, as there is no effective medical treatment available. Cataract is not a growth; once removed, it cannot recur. Once the lens is removed, it is replaced with an artificial lens inserted into the pocket formed by the original lens capsule that remains in the eye.

Diagnosis of cataract involves systemic and ophthalmic examination together with electroretinography and ultrasound if possible, to determine presence of other ocular diseases and to assess the integrity and functionality of retina.

Replacement of intraocular lenses has been used following cataract removal in humans since the 1950s. Intra ocular lens in animals was thought by many veterinary surgeons too. First such attempt was made as back as 1956. Initially, the human lenses were tried out for the dog but recent work has proven that it needs special lenses in dogs to achieve acuity and a better vision. In animal patients where glasses or contacts are impractical, the need for intraocular correction is even greater.

In humans, a lens of 16-18 diopters (D) is generally used. Measurements in dog eyes indicate that a lens of 40-43D is required. Intraocular lenses are most often made of an optical portion of polymethylmethacrylate (PMMA) with flexible haptics to fix the lens within the capsular bag. Complications following intraocular lens implantation are uncommon and not usually associated with the presence of the replacement lens itself.

The success rate of cataract surgeries has risen significantly during the recent decades, especially due to the development of phacoemulsification and intra ocular lens (IOL) implantation (3,4).However, there are only few institutes in India that are fully equipped with essential equipment and have trained veterinary ophthalmologist to carry out the diagnostic procedures and manage the ocular affections. This compilation is aimed to develop awareness among vets and pet owners in regard with Cataract surgery.

2

Cataract- An Overview

(A) Anatomy of Lens

The lens is anoptically clear, avascular, biconvex structure of crystalline appearance with an anterior surfaceless curved than the posterior surface, placed between the iris and the vitreous. It is suspended by the suspensory ligament of the lens which is attached to the ciliary body and equator of the lens.

The lens consists of a central nucleus surrounded by the lens fibres and anterior epithelium, encapsulated in an elastic lens capsule. The anterior surface of the lens is in contact with the posterior surface of the iris whereas posterior surface is in contact with the vitreous. As the adult lens does not have a blood supply, its metabolic needs are met by the aqueous humour.The lens is composed of 65% water, 35% protein with scant amounts of electrolytes. The proteins can besubdivided into soluble proteins, or crystalline, and insoluble, or albuminoid, proteins (5). The lens acts as a refractive media and allows unaltered passage of light and images to the retina.

Of the approximately 60 D of total refractive power of the eye, the lens contributes approximately 13–16 D in humans and approximately 40 D in dogs. Dog a have a very short accommodative power of 1-2 D as compared with that of 2-8 D in cats and 9-14 D in humans in respect with age. Lens accounts for 30%-35% of the eye's refractive power and is used for fine refractive adjustment and for focusing on objects at different distances (5).

(B) Definition of Cataract

The term cataract comprises a common group of ocular disorders manifested as loss of transparency of the lens or its capsule. The opacities may be of varying sizes, shapes, location within the lens depending upon etiology, age of onset, and rate of progression (6). Opacification of its fibers and alteration in water content are the only pathologic changes the lens can undergo, since it is devoid of blood supply after birth. Unlike other tissues, it cannot react to deleterious physical and chemical agents by an inflammatory or allergic process (7).Cataracts or opacities of the lens of the eye are a leading cause of blindness or an increasing cause of vision loss in dogs (8).

(C) Incidence of Cataract

Wide variety in incidence of cataract has been recorded in studies. This could be attributed to thepopulation variance of breed in the particular region.

Incidence of familial, congenital, or neonatal cataracts are seen in German shepherd dog, Golden Retriever, West Highland white terrier, and the Pembroke Welsh Corgi,Bichon Frise, Cocker Spaniel, Boston terrier, Miniature Schnauzer (9,10).

Prevalence of cataracts in the general canine population increases with age and by the age of 13.5 years usually all the dogs develop some degree of lens opacity (11).

Highest incidence of cataract in dogs is seen more in the age group of 7-15 years followed by 0-3 year age group dogs and 3-7 years age group. Regarding breed wise the incidence of cataract was highest in Spitz (36.49%), followed by non-descript (21.8%), Labrador (14.2%), German shepherd (6.06%), Cocker Spaniel and Rottweiler (5.2%) and Terrier (3.3%) and other breeds (3.78%). The incidence was more in males than in females in all the breeds (12).

(D) Causes of Cataract

There are numerous potential causes for cataracts, including metabolism (diabetes), nutrition (use of milk replacers), developmental ocular defects, trauma, etc. However, the most common cause of cataracts in dogs appears to be genetic disposition. Senility is probably another major cause of canine cataracts, though the exact prevalence (and causes) of age-related cataracts in dogs remains unknown (13).

Several toxic substances can produce cataractous lenticular changes when administered systematically. Certain hydrocarbons or substituted hydrocarbons (Naphthalene and Dinitrophenol), salts of certain metals (Thallium. Cobalt, Selenium), antimitotic agents, enzyme inhibitors and number of drugs causes lenticular cataract (14).

Severe trauma to the globe due to crushing non-penetrating blow from impact with an automobile can also cause cataracts (15).

Deficiency of amino acids and vitamins in diet may lead to cataract. The absence of tryptophan may lead to abnormal maturation of lens fibers so that cell nuclei do not disappear but are replaced by small densely staining particles (16).

There are numerous theories as the cause of cataract. These include; Oxidative damage caused by oxygen free radicals (hydroxyl ions, hydrogen peroxide and ultraviolet radiation). Deficiency of antioxidants like glutathione, catalase and ascorbate can result into cataractogenic changes in the lens. As the lens ages the insoluble protein content in the lens increases more than the soluble protein, which eventually leads to cataract development. Electrolyte disturbances like increase in Na^+ and Ca^{++} ion levels and decrease in K^+ ions within lens due to decreased activity of Na^+ / K^+ adenosine triphosphate pump in epithelium may lead to development of cataract within the lens (17).

Chronic anterior uveitis can lead to cataract formation by altering the aqueous humour, which subsequently affects lens nutrition. The majority of uveitis induced cataracts are inoperable because of inflammation-induced intraocular tissue changes, such as synechia, secondary glaucoma, and preiridial fibro vascular membranes (18).

(E) Pathogenesis of Cataract

The exact biochemical disorders responsible for the formation of cataracts in domestic animals are not perfectly understood. However, in general it may be stated that noxious influences affecting lens nutrition, energy metabolism, protein metabolism and osmotic balance may result in opacity. Once these disturbances occur, they will cause irreversible changes in lens protein contents, metabolic pumps, ionic concentrations, and antioxidant activity.

The proportion of insoluble (albuminoid) proteins in the lens increases at the expense of the soluble (crystallin) protein fraction. Epithelial Na^+/K^+ adenosine triphosphate pump activity decreases, resulting in a shift in the ionic balance within the lens, and antioxidant activity in the lens likewise diminishes. At the same time, proteolytic enzyme activity increases in the lens, causing breakdown of cell membranes and degradation of lens protein. All of these events amplify and cascade as the cataract progresses, causing visible changes in the lens. These changes are caused by morphologic changes in the lens capsule, epithelium, and fibers that accompany the molecular events. The end result is loss of transparency due to lens fibers rupture, cell death, and water-cleft formation (5).

The avascular lens of the eye is freely permeable to glucose, its main energy source. Glucose enters by diffusion from the surrounding aqueous humor, which is an ultrafiltrate of plasma. Normally, most glucose is then converted to lactic acid via the anaerobic glycolytic path way. Lactic acid diffuses back out of the lens and into circulation. However, when there is persistent hyperglycemia, the hexokinase enzyme responsible for this conversion becomes saturated.

Excess glucose then gets metabolized through the polyol pathway to sorbitol and fructose, which are not freely diffusible. Sorbitol and fructose, which are trapped in the lens, act as hydrophilic osmotic agents, drawing water into the lens and causing swelling and rupture of lens fibers, resulting in the lenticular opacities known as cataracts (19).

(F) Classification of Cataract

A thorough medical history and complete physical examination preceding a thorough ophthalmic examination is essential for proper classification of cataract. Cataract may be classified by numerous methods including location, age of onset, cause, and degree of maturation. Each method has its advantage and limitations, therefore all are used simultaneously to accurately describe a cataractous lens. Classification is also used to assist in predicting the associated loss of vision and anticipated progression of the cataract.

1. Age of onset

The age of onset helps in determining the cause and is particularly characteristic for the inherited cataract in certain breeds as it is often distributed. The different types are given below;

i. ***Congenital cataract:*** Congenital cataract is present at the time of birth. It is often nuclear and sometimes both nuclear and cortical (20). Most congenital cataracts are bilateral (21) and remains stationary for life and do not cause visual impairment. It may be of maternal origin resulting from infectious or toxic agent (22).

ii. ***Juvenile or developmental or early onset cataract:*** This type of cataract develops during early years of life (< 6 years of age). Juvenile cataracts are hereditary in many breeds e.g. Afghan hound and Standard Poodle (23). The other non-inherited causes include trauma, diabetes, intraocular inflammation and toxicity.

iii. ***Senile or late onset or senescent cataract:*** Develop in dogs over 6 years of age. Senile cataracts are simply associated with advancement of age. It may affect the nucleus as well as the cortex. They are typically classified as senile if no other antecedent etiology is known or apparent. Prevalence of cataracts in the general canine population increases with age and by the age of 13.5 years all dogs develop some degree of lens opacity (11).

2. Stage of maturation

Stage of maturation refers to the appearance of lens regardless of age of animal or the underlying problem causing cataract(24). Not all the cataract progresses through each stage of maturation. Stage of maturation has been considered important while determining whether a dog is a candidate for surgery. The different types are given below:

i. ***Incipient cataract*:** This cataract represents very early lenticular changes and is not associated with visual impairment. Usually less than 15% of lens is opaque.

ii. ***Immature cataract:*** This stage is quite variable in its presentation. 10-99% of lens may be affected but tapetal reflection will be present through some portion of lens. Vision may be impaired to a variable extent but as the cataract progresses to maturity, vision may be absent.

iii. ***Mature cataract*:** In this stage there will be total or solid opacification of lens and absence of tapetal reflection making the animal functionally blind. Normal lenticular size and absence of fundic reflex are other characters of mature cataract.

iv. ***Intumescent cataract*:** In this stage the lens may become markedly increased in size due to imbibition of fluid. This enlargement of lens leads to the splitting and separation of the lens suture lines with the resultant Y shaped fissure. Imbibition of fluid may be quite rapid resulting in complete opacification. Vision may be impaired to a variable extent.

v. ***Hypermature cataract*:** In this stage some of the lens fibers undergo liquefaction. Occasionally during liquefaction of the cortex diffusion of liquefied cortical material across the apparently intact lens capsule may occur. Leaking of liquefied cortical material from the hypermature cataract result in a variable iridocyclitis. It occurs because lens protein is immunologically foreign to the animal's immune system.

vi. ***Morgagnian cataract*:** Here there is liquefaction of cortex with an intact nucleus. The nucleus may drop or sink ventrally to the bottom of the capsular bag when the cortex liquefies.

3. Depending upon causes

It is one of the most important and useful classification of cataract.

i. ***Inherited Cataracts:*** A large number of cataracts in the purebred dog population have an inherited basis. Diagnosis and management of inherited cataracts is important to check its transmission in the general population. The mode of inheritance included both dominant and recessive pattern in dogs(25).

ii. ***Traumatic cataract:*** Trauma resulting from crushing, non-penetrating blow from impact with an automobile leading to tearing of anterior capsule or dis-insertion of the zonular ligaments may cause traumatic cataract. With tearing of the lens capsule, lens protein material which is foreign to the immune system, leaks into the anterior chamber leading to an inflammatory response (15).

iii. ***Metabolic cataract:*** Many metabolic disorders like diabetes and hypocalcaemia result in defective lens nourishment which in turn leads to cataract. Diabetic cataracts frequently develop rapidly and progress to maturity. Early surgical removal of diabetic cataracts usually carries a similar success rate to that of non-diabetic cataracts, so long as the medical complications due to diabetes are controlled and the animal is well stabilized on insulin prior to surgery (26). Clinically, diabetic cataracts tend to develop bilaterally and at a rapid rate (27).

    Hypocalcaemia associated with parathyroid dysfunction, post parturient hypocalcaemia, and severe nutritional imbalances in the young animal produces characteristic multifocal anterior and posterior cortical opacities (28). The mechanism is probably through alterations of lens cell membrane permeability from altered extracellular levels of calcium (29).

iv. ***Complicated or secondary cataracts:*** Ocular injury, uveitis or other intraocular inflammation and some systemic illnesses may result in cataract (30). If there is minor damage to the lens and the cause is ameliorated, the opacity formed probably will be stationary. If there is recurrent uveitis or if the original injury severely damaged the lens, the opacity may enlarge and eventually involve the entire lens.

v. ***Toxic cataract:*** Numerous drugs will cause lenticular opacities (31). Fortunately, most of the common therapeutic agents do not appear to be cataractogenic in the normally used doses. Disophenol, used in treating hookworm infection, can cause lenticular opacities at doses not much higher than used clinically, but these opacities usually are reversible after the drug is discontinued (32,33).

4. *Location within the lens* (34)

The cataractous process may be confined to a single area within the lens and its capsule or may affect the entire structure.

i. ***Capsular cataract:*** Opacity confined to the lens capsule.

ii. ***Subcapsular cataract:*** In this opacity involves cortex immediately beneath the lens capsule. It usually affects the back of lens and progress more quickly than other type. Subcapsular cataracts cause blurriness and glare.

iii. ***Cortical cataract:*** Spot like opacities or cuneiform cataracts appearing in the lens's outer rim and extending "spokes" towards the central core. These spokes block light, causing glare and loss of contrast. Both near and distance visions are slowly disrupted. Diabetics often develop this type of cataract.

iv. ***Nuclear cataract:*** These are the most common cataract, typically known as "age-related cataract." Found in the center of the lens, they interfere with the ability to see distant.

3

Diagnosis of Cataract

The speed with which changes in the eye can take place is challenging. Ophthalmic problems do not lend themselves to casual examination or 'trial and error' therapy. Therefore, to perform safe cataract surgery with good quality outcome, uniform minimum standard of diagnostic and clinical practice needed to be in place.

Although cataract can be diagnosed by routine gross examination of the affected dog even then it is mandatary to develop a routine ophthalmic examinations in a consistent and organized manner to make a confirmatory diagnosis and plan the surgical technique for a favourable prognosis. A sequential examination starting right from history up to electroretinography may be performed as under:

History » Gross Examination » Menace response test » Obstacle course test » dazzle or photic blink reflex » Light induced pupillary reflexes (direct/ consensual) » Corneal reflex test »Schirmer's tear test»Fluorescein dye test » Tonometry » Ultrasonographical examination » Fundus examination (Direct and Indirect Ophthalmoscopy) » Electroretinography.

Diagnostic Kit: It consisted of essential diagnostic equipments and eye solutions which are used for detailed ophthalmic examination. These include direct ophthalmoscope, head mounted indirect binocular ophthalmoscope with 20 D lens, Tonometer, ERG unit, USG machine with 5-14MHZ linear array probe, fluorescein dye strips, Schirmer's tear test strip, mydriatic agent Tropicamide, Coupling gel for USG and Viscomet for ERG.

***History of Patient*:** The Information regarding animal's breed, age, sex, general health, vision status, duration of the blindness, probable history of any injury, history pertaining to visual activity during the day and night, signs of vision impairment (bumping into walls or other objects, tripping, misjudging distances, not recognizing familiar people), increased intake of water and increased frequency of urination in dogs suspected with *diabetes mellitus* and details of previous medical record are to be obtained and analysed during detailed ophthalmological examination.

***Gross Examinations*:** The affected eyes should be checked for clarity of cornea, opacity of lens, type of cataract, conjunctival appearance, conjunctival vascularity and discharge, if any.

Detailed Ophthalmic Examinations

The purpose of the diagnostic protocol is to confirm the diagnosis of visually significant cataract, to ensure that cataract is the cause of the visual symptoms and to determine if there is any co-existing ocular pathology.

Complete ophthalmic examination of the affected eyes should bedone with the help of visual function tests, tonometry, direct and indirect ophthalmoscopy, ocular ultrasonography and ERG.

***Visual function Tests*:** (*Adopted from 35, 36*)

1. ***Menace reflex test (Fig.1)*:** - It is performed by moving one hand swiftly toward the dog's face, then stopping abruptly taking care not to touch the vibrissae and checking for a blink reaction. A positive blink reaction leads to reflex closure of palpebral fissure and turning of head away from the stimulus.

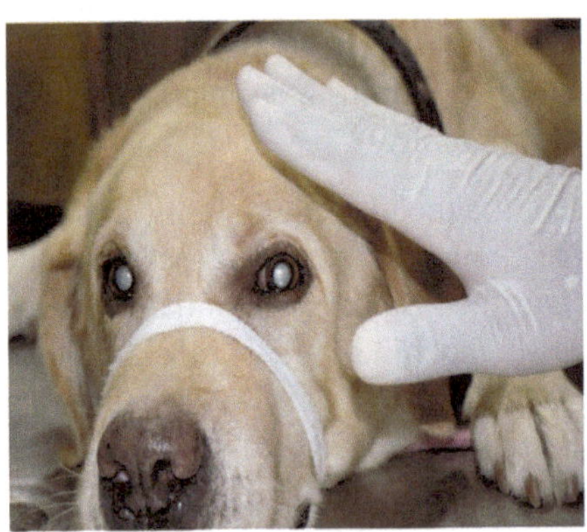
Negative

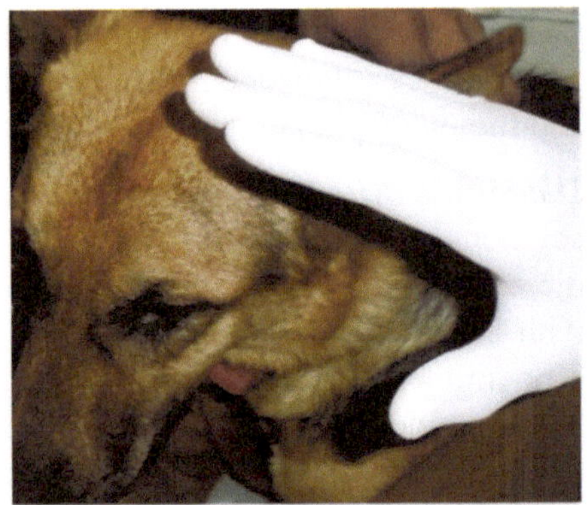
Positive

Fig. 1: Menace reflex test performed to check blink reaction

2. ***Corneal reflex test (Fig.2):*** - It is done by touching a wisp of cotton wool to the lateral region of the cornea (i.e. away from the visual axis), a blink response was considered as a positive corneal reflex.

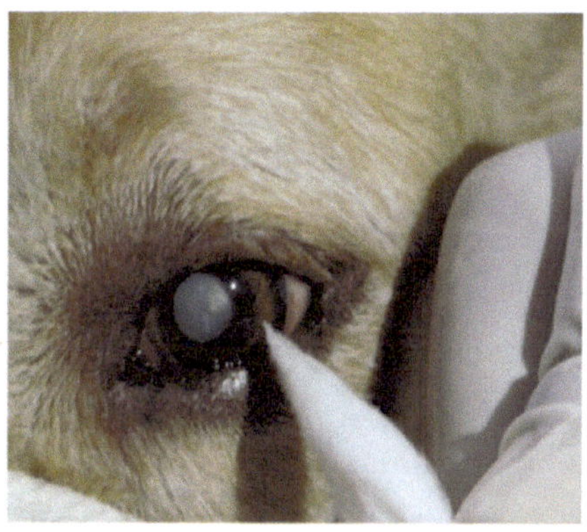

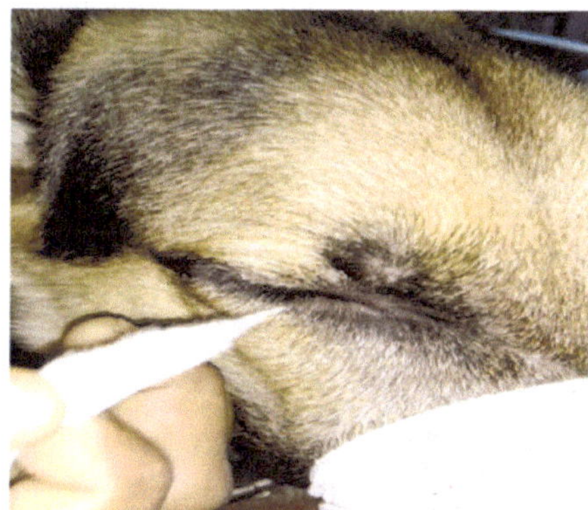

Negative Positive

Fig. 2: Corneal reflex test

3. ***Light Induced Pupillary Reflexes (Fig. 3):*** - Also called as pupillary light reflex (PLR). The penlight or torch is moved back and forth between both pupils (swinging flashlight test) to create dynamic contraction (anisocoria), the pupil under the direct light stimulation would be slightly smaller than the opposite consensual pupil size. This is considered as normal or satisfactory pupillary reflex.

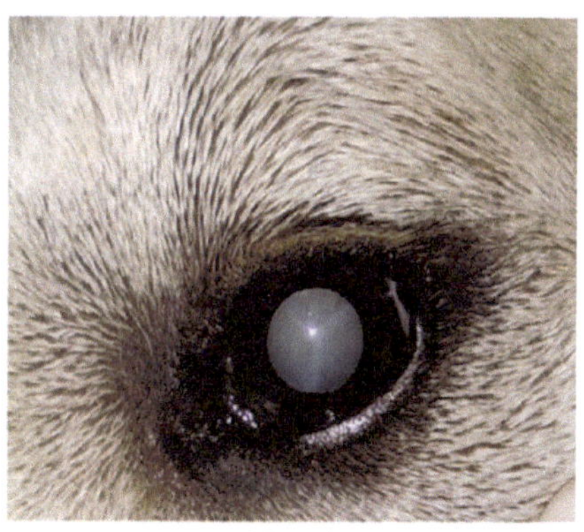

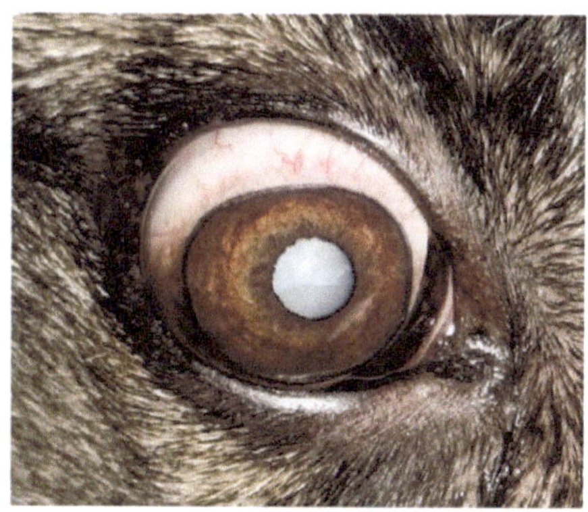

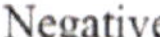

Negative Positive

Fig. 3: Pupillary light reflexes test

4. ***Dazzle or Photic Blink Reflex (Fig. 4)**:* This test is performed by focusing a direct beam of bright light at the ocular fundus. A positive reflex is manifested as a bilateral partial blink response to the bright light.

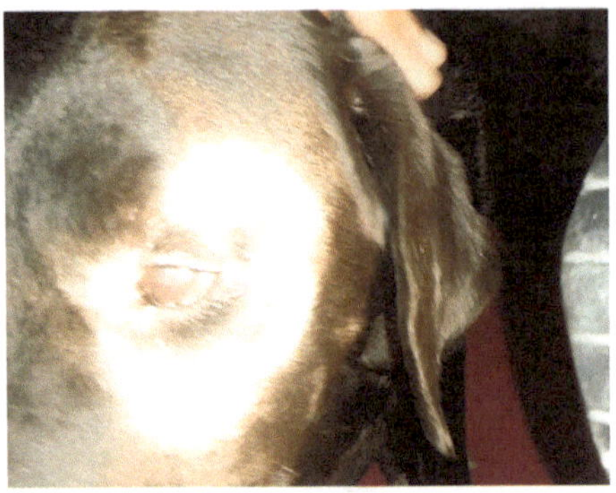

Negative

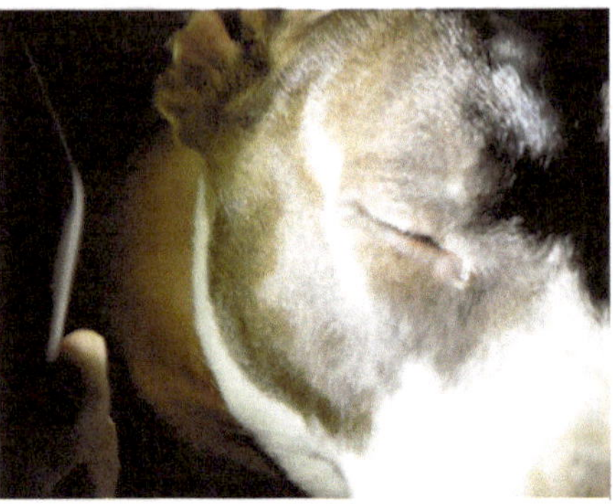

Positive

Fig. 4: *Dazzle Reflex* Test performed by focusing bright light at ocular fundus

5. ***Obstacle course test (Fig. 5):*** -The animal is evaluated for its movements in normal and dim light. The animals with significant visual deficits that fail in the obstacles test will demonstrate an altered or accentuated gait, or simply refuse to move.

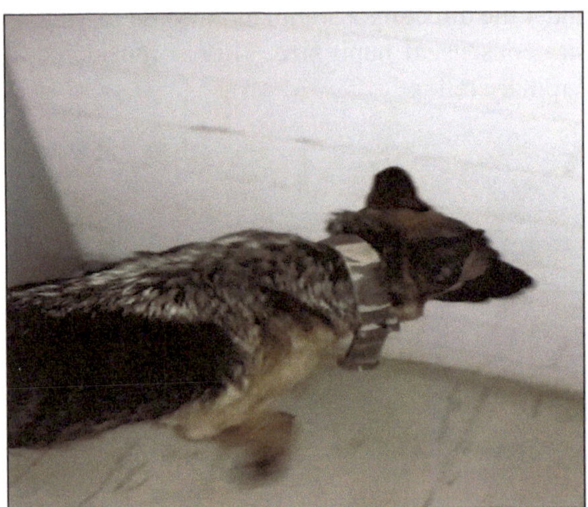

Nagative obstacke course (Dog bumping into wall)

Fig. 5: Obstacle Course test conducted to determine significant visual defects

6. ***Schirmer's Tear Test (Fig. 6):*** Itis performed to measure the tear production, using sterile diagnostic strips (5mm 40mm). These strips are readily available in market. The Schirmer tear strip is placed in the medioventral to lateral third of the palpebral conjunctival fornix for one minute. The strip is removed from the eye and tear wetting is compared to millimeter scale. The value is graded as normal (15-25mm/min).

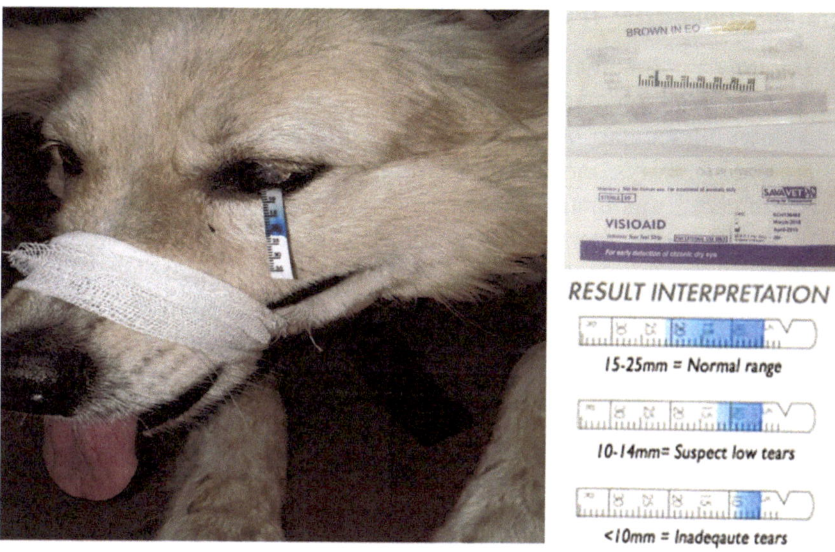

Fig. 6: Schirmer Tear Test performed to test tear production by using a diagnostic strip

7. ***Fluorescein Dye Test (Fig. 7):*** It is performed to evaluate ulcers and epithelial defects in cornea. The Fluorescein sodium ophthalmic strip is moistened with sterile saline and then placed in the palpebral fissure. After 5 minutes, the strip is removed and the excess stain is washed out using normal saline. The visualisation of fluorescein stain is enhanced by a cobalt blue light.

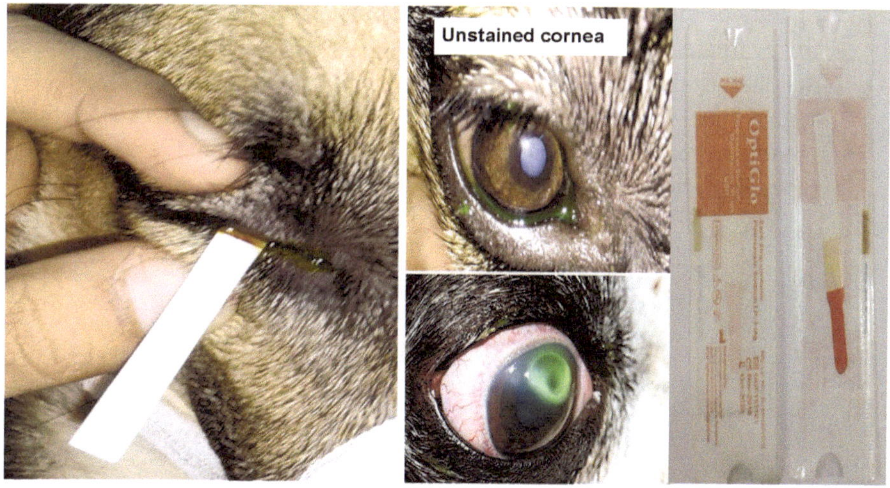

Stained corneal ulcer

Fig. 7: Fluorescein Dye Test performed to diagnose ulcers or epithelial defects of cornea

***Additional Diagnostic Test*: (Adopted from 37and 38)**

1. ***Tonometry*:** Tonometry is the measurement of intraocular pressure. Abnormal intraocular pressures can indicate subtle disease processes. A low intraocular pressure usually indicates anterior uveitis. High pressures always indicate glaucoma (39). Although studies showed Significant tonometric differences between the immature and hypermature cataract groups, but these differences are too small to be clinically useful Decreased intraocular pressure of dogs with all stages of cataract formation suggests concurrent lens induced uveitis during all stages of cataract formation, especially with the mature and hypermature stages. There are different methods with different working principle for measurement of IOP in dogs such as Applanation, Indentation and Rebound tonometry. Although significant variation is recorded among individuals as well as among techniques and the time of the day at which IOP is measured even than the approximately reported normal IOP range is 10-20 mm Hg (40).

   A significant decrease in the mature and hypermature cataractous eyes may be found as compared to the incipient and immature groups indicating lens induced uveitis (LIU) which has a tendency to increase with cataract progression as indicated on analysis of clinical signs of uveitis (41).

2. ***Ultrasonographical examination (Fig. 9&10)*:** Ultrasongraphic examination could detect abnormalities of the posterior segment when opacity of the anterior segment hinders the ophthalmologic examinations to evaluate the posterior segment for complications like vitreal degeneration and retinal detachment or optic disc cupping (42,43) and with respect to the selection of patient for cataract removal (40). Patients having increased echogenicity of the normally anechoic lens without any other posterior segment complications results in favourable prognosis.

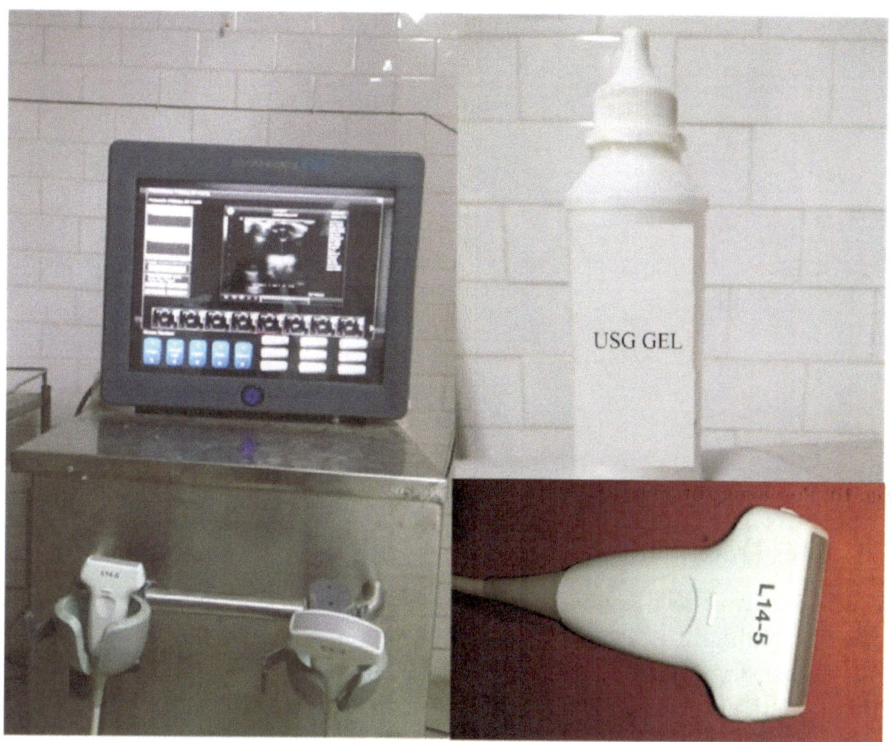

Fig. 9: Ocular Ultrasonography **A.** Monitor, **B.** Gel, **C.** Transducer

Ophthalmic ultrasonography is performed with an ultrasound frequencies ranging from 7.5 to 50 MHz to evaluate intraocular and retro-bulbar tissues with or without sedation. The examination is performed in lateral recumbency. Eye lids are held open manually (Fig. 10). Transducer is directly placed on the cornea after application of coupling gel. Scanning depth is kept 4 cm while frequency isset to 14 MHz. After ultrasound examination, excess coupling gel is carefully wiped from the eyes and rinsed with sterile 0.9% sodium chloride solution to prevent the corneal irritation and eyes are re-examined for the identification and treatment, if necessary, of iatrogenic corneal lesions resulting from the examination. The globes are examined in a sagittal (longitudinal) plane.

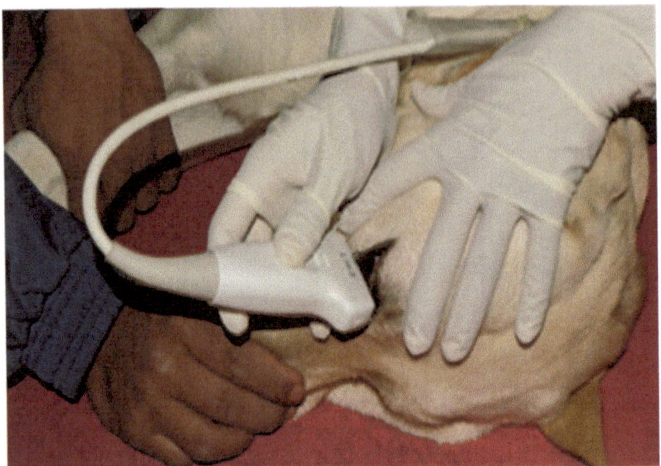

Fig. 10: Positioning of probe for Ocular USG of a dog

3. Fundus Examination

The easiest way to diagnose a cataract is to visualise it against the tapetal reflex. To highlight a cataract against a tapetal reflex it is best to look at it from a distance using a bright focal light source. A simple and useful technique is distant ophthalmoscopy. Any opacity in the visual axis will cast a shadow and appear black against the bright tapetal reflex (1).

Examination of fundus depends on the stage of the cataract. In case of incipient or early immature cataracts, fundus is not completely obscured and ophthalmoscopy is possible for fundus examination through the lens to evaluate the retina. However, this isn't possible with a mature or hypermature cataract. In advanced cases of hypermature cataract where cortical lens is resorbed tapetal reflex may be seen by focused retro-illumination. Direct and Indirect ophthalmoscopy is useful to assess the clarity of the cornea, determine the position of opacities within the lens, differentiate nuclear cataract from nuclear sclerosis, assess the stage of cataract, position of the cataractous lens (luxation or sublxation) etc.

Both, direct and indirect ophthalmoscopy is done after achieving mydriasis by instillation of topical 1% tropicamide 20 minutes prior to examination.

A. ***Direct Ophthalmoscope (Fig. 11):*** The dog is kept in seated position facing the examiner with one hand under the muzzle and the eyelids are kept apart with another hand. The ophthalmoscope is kept very close to the observer's eye. The tapetal reflex, if present,would be visible from a distance of about 50 cm from the patient. After alignment of image the observer and instrument should move forward until the instrument is close to the dog's cornea. In case of incipient and early immature cataracts the, if possible, optic nerve head is identified and examined, followed by the rest of the tapetal and non tapetal fundus in quadrants.

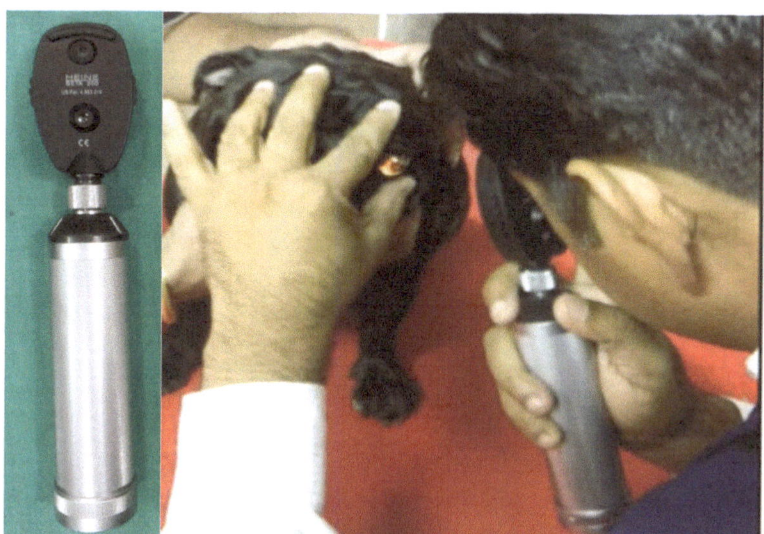

Fig. 11: Ophthalmoscopy Direct

B. ***Indirect Binocular Ophthalmoscopy (Fig.12):*** This technique allows a larger view of examination of a cataractous eye from a greater and safer working distance from the dog. It is done with the help of a head mounted indirect ophthalmoscope placing a +20 D double aspheric glass optics between the dog's and the examiner's eyes.

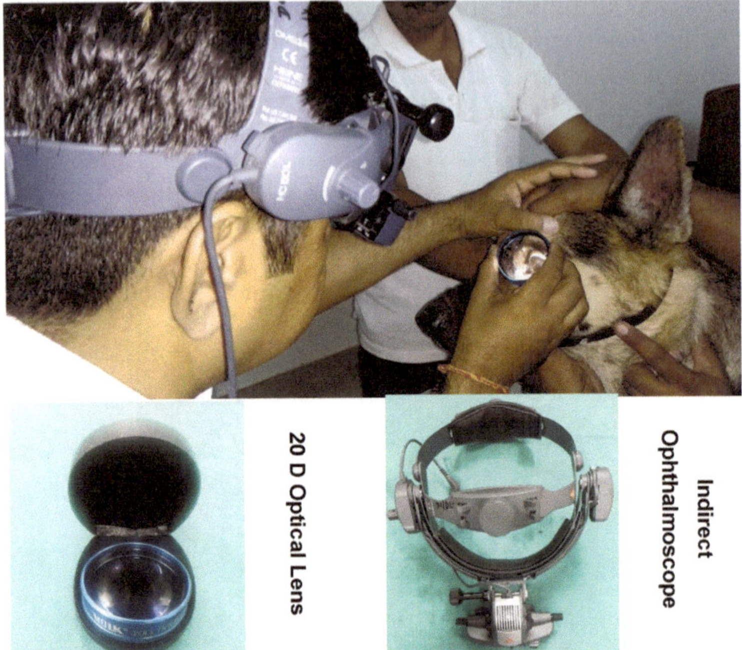

Fig. 12: Indirect Ophthalmoscopy

4 *Electroretinography* (Fig. 13)

Preoperative electroretinography (ERG) using HMsERG (Hand held multispecies Electroretinography) unit helps to evaluate retinal functions in cataractous eyes after application of topical 1 tropicamide for maximal pupillary dilation as mydriatic (2 drops every 10 minutes) and 0.5 Povidine Iodine for ocular antisepsis 2-3 times, 30 minutes prior to procedure.

ERG is performed under general anaesthesia. An adequate amount of gel Hypromellose Ophthalmic Solution is applied on the inner surface of the Koijman electrode before using it on the cornea.Various steps of ERGareperformed in a closed room securing the dog in sternal recumbency and cotton pillow is used to elevate and position the head. Two Needle electrodes are used as reference and ground electrode. A reference electrode (black cable) is placed subcutaneously halfway between the temporal canthus and the ear. A similar subcutaneous ground electrode (blue) is placed at an indifferent position i.e. at the central top portion of the head. The active electrode is placed directly on the cornea after topical anaesthesia with 0.5% proparacaine. An adequate amount of gel hypromellose ophthalmic solution is applied on the inner surface of the Koijman electrode before using it on the cornea. Scotopic (rod and combined rod-cone) and Photopic (cone and 30-Hz response) flicker LED programme is selected in the HMsERG system for a quick ERG recording and the photopic and scotopic vision is tested with a standard flash (3.0 cd. s/m2). Electroretinographs are recorded automatically and the a- and b- wave amplitude (μV), and implicitctime (ms) are auto generated using the dog diagnostic protocol pre-programmed for this equipment (44).

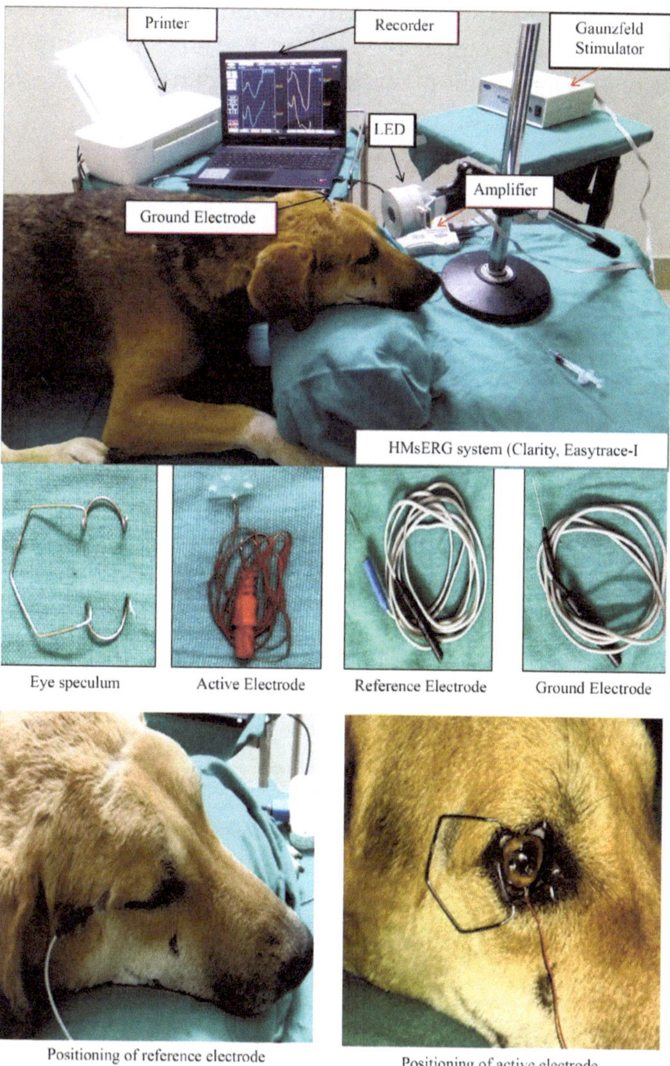

Fig. 13: ERG (Instrumentation and positloning

3. ***Haemato-biochemical examination*:** Haematological examination and blood biochemistry (Serum creatinine, BUN, ALT, AST, ALKP and Blood glucose) are estimated to rule out any concomitant disease or diabetes as a cause for cataract.

Diabetic animals frequently develop cataracts but can also have numerous other ocular problems, including uveitis, keratopathy, retinopathy, and the effects of lipid derangements and systemic hypertension. As part of the diffuse neuropathy affecting the sensorimotor nervous system of diabetics, corneal sensation may be decreased and result in or complicate recurrent or indolent corneal ulcer (45).

4

Selection of Patient for Cataract Surgery

All animals with cataract are not suitable candidates for surgery. Pre-surgical assessment of a candidate is essential to make a safe judgement for surgical procedure to perform lensectomy. Failure in canine cataract surgery can be associated with poor case selection. A thorough ocular and physical examination should be performed to rule out other ocular diseases prior to cataract surgery. The cataractous lenses in both eyes must be mature to cause functional loss of vision. (24).

The following prerequisites should be fulfilled before cataract extraction is recommended (6):

1. The affected eye should have a significant visual deficit.
2. For the patient to regain vision, its retina must be healthy and functional. if the fundus cannot be examined thoroughly (because of the cataract), retinal function should be evaluated with electroretinography (ERG) to ensure that retinal degeneration is not present as the patient history, signalment, and the speed of pupil contraction in response to light are not reliable indicators of the presence or absence of progressive rod-cone degeneration.
3. Any incipient LIU—indicated by ciliary injection, hypotony, miosis, aqueous flare, change in iris color, or resistance to mydriasis—must first be controlled by topical corticosteroids and/or NSAIDs. The incidence of short- and long-term complications is greater when uveitis is present preoperatively.
4. No other ocular pathologic process should be present. In many practices an ultrasound examination is performed before surgery to rule out vitreal/retinal detachment.
5. The patient should be in good general health, should not suffer from any systemic diseases, and should undergo tests to ensure it is a suitable candidate for anesthesia.

6. The patient must be amenable to intensive handling, because frequent topical applications of medication are required in both the preoperative and postoperative periods.

Selection of patient for cataract surgery plays a vital role in the outcome. Assessment of the patient begins with a medical and visual history, including a physical examination and laboratory diagnostics to rule out systemic diseases, such as *diabetes mellitus*, that may contribute to cataract formation. Neurological evaluation and behavior assessment are essential in ruling out age-related changes in mentation, activity level or cognitive dysfunction that may be misinterpreted as a decline in vision. Aggressive or unruly patients may not be candidates for surgery due to the inability to consistently provide medical therapy that will be needed both preoperatively and postoperatively. The history is important to determine the progression of visual deficit; eg. nyctalopia (night blindness) is often a sign of retinal degeneration (46).

A Schirmer's tear test should always be done before cataract surgery. The normal tear production rate is 15 to 25 mm/min. A rate below 10 mm/min with concurrent conjunctivitis, corneal pigmentation, neovascularisation, and scarring indicates the presence of keratoconjunctivitis sicca, a syndrome of decreased tear production. Surgery may still be possible when tear production is low if production can be increased by using topical cyclosporine and if the cornea is not scarred. A borderline tear production rate (12 to 14 mm/min) should be rechecked just before surgery. If borderline tear production exists, the ophthalmologist may elect to use cyclosporine before surgery to increase tear production to a normal level or may elect to treat the dog with artificial tear ointments in the immediate postoperative period (47).

5

Surgical Management of Cataract

Good cataract outcome depends on pre-operative selection of patients, the skills and knowledge of the eye surgeon, the surgical technique, the surgical facilities and environment, the post-operative care and the optical correction provided.

Preoperative Procedures

Owners are advised to instill antibiotic eye drop such as Moxifloxacin @ two drops b.i.d. for 7 days and eye drop tropicamide @ two drops b.i.d. for 2 days before the cataract surgery for proper dilation of pupil. Non-steroidal anti-inflammatory eye drops such as Flubriprofenis started t.i.d on the day before surgery. Further, tropicamide (1%) used as mydriatic agent is instilled 30 minutes before operation at the rate of two drops every 5 minutes in the eye to be operated. 0.5% povidone iodine drops are instilled on cornea prior to surgery.

Anaesthesia

The cataract surgery is performed under general anaesthesia, be it injectable like ketamine or gaseous like Isoflurane. Additionally, retrobulbar nerve block may be achieved by depositing 3 ml of 2% lignocainebehind the globe at orbital stalk by palpating ventral orbital rim.

Ophthalmological Instruments (Fig.17)

A	Corneal scissors	B and C	Tying forceps (curved)
D	Tying forceps (straight)	E	Needle holder
F	Halsted mosquito forceps (straight)	G	Halsted Mosquito Forceps (curved)
H	Wire eyelid speculum	I	Keratome 2.8 mm
J	15^0 Lance tip blade	K	Utrata capsulorrhexis forceps (angled)
L and M	Utrata capsulorrhexis forceps (pointed tip)	N	Corneal forceps
O	Phaco pre chopper	P	Nucleus rotator
Q	Sinskey lens hook, angled	R	Castroviejo needle holder
S	Bard-Parker handle no.3	T	Mayo scissors (straight)

Ophthalmic Disposables

1	Eye dress	2	Viscoelastic	3	Vicryl 10/0 absorbable suture material
4	Silk thread no.1	5	Elizabethan Collar		

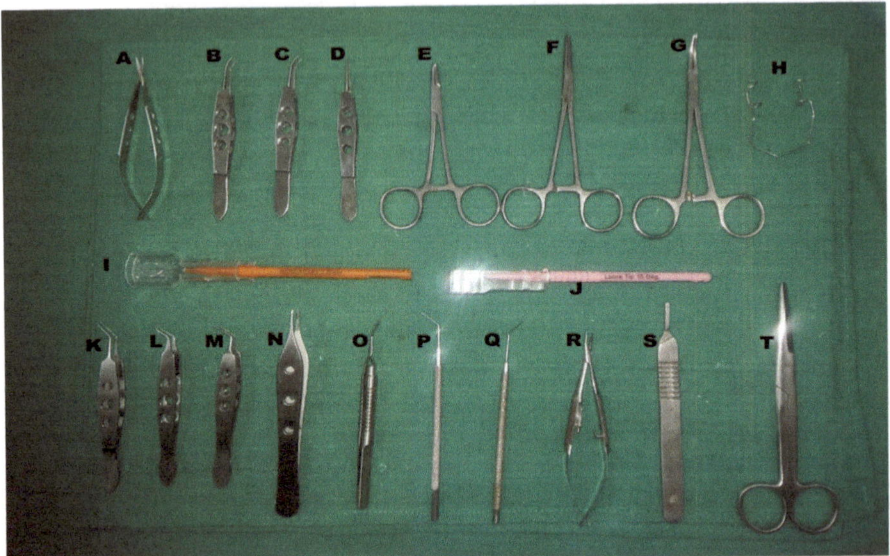

Fig. 17: Ophthalmic Surgery Instruments

Operative Procedure

The different procedures to remove cataracts in dogs are:

- Intracapsular extraction of lens (ICCE)
- Extracapsular extraction of lens (ECCE)
- Phacoemulsification of cataractous lens

Intracapsular extraction of lens (ICCE)

The intracapsular extraction technique is rarely used for cataract removal because of its hazards, more risks and the lowest success rates. However, removal of subluxated lenses, anterior luxated lenses, and posterior luxated (intravitreal) lenses uses the intracapsular technique in which the entire cataractous lens is removed without opening the lens capsule. This technique is particularly used to remove the luxated lenses, following tearing of the zonules. It has become obsolete nowadays.

Extracapsular extraction of lens (ECCE): (Fig.18)

The extracapsular procedure, used in the dog in the 1960s through the early 1980s, has been largely replaced by phacoemulsification. Extracapsular cataract extraction can be done by using magnifying loupe, table mounted microscope and with advancement it can be more safely done by using operative microscope. It involves a 180-degree incision in the peripheral cornea with removal of the anterior lens capsule and manual expression of the lens cortex and nucleus. This technique is necessary in the removal of very dense cataracts.

Corneal incision is closed with 8/0 absorbable suture material using simple interrupted suture. The sutures are placed one mm apart and knots are rotated on the scleral side. Anterior chamber is re-inflated by injecting air into the chamber. After completion of the surgery subconjuctival injection of Gentamicin (0.5 ml) + Dexamethasone (0.5 ml) is given using 24 G needle. Temporary tarsorrhaphy is performed by horizontal mattress suture to protect the eye.

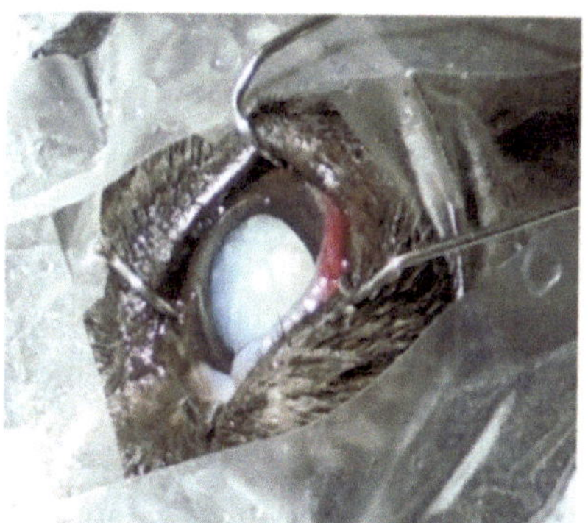

Fig.18(a). Position of the eye under operating microscope

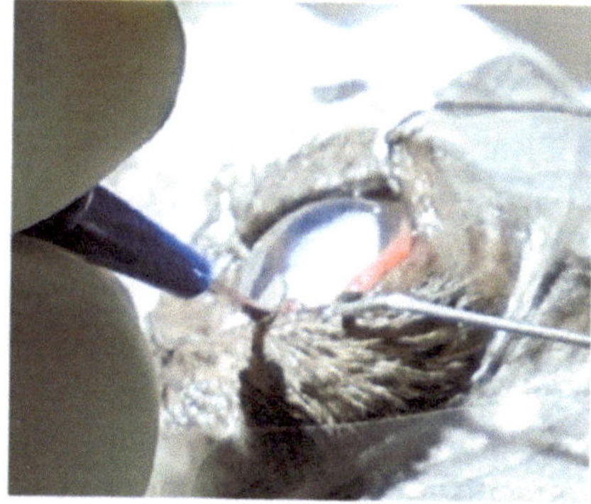

Fig.18(b). Incision on cornea with Keratotome

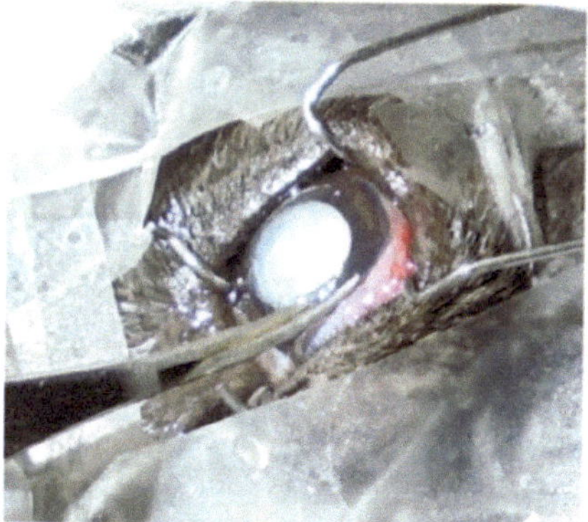

Fig. 18 (c). Enlargement of corneal incision for smooth delivery of lens

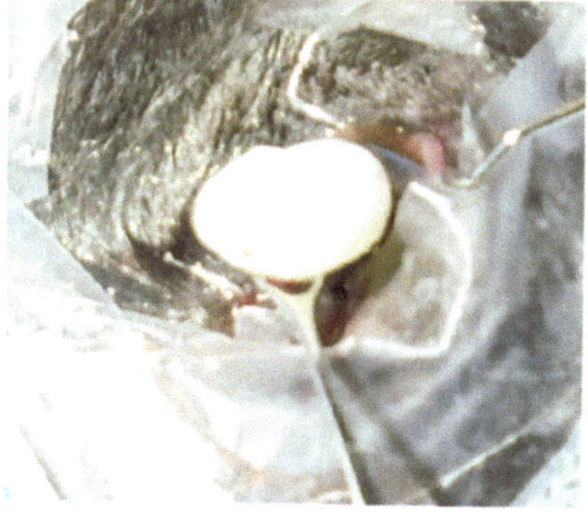

Fig. 18 (d). Removal of mature cataractous lens

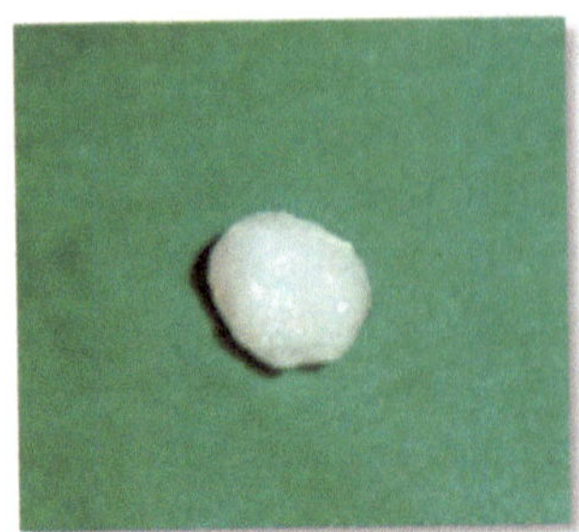

Fig. 18(e). Surgical Procedure of Extracapsular Cataract Extraction (ECCE) Method

Phacoemulsification of cataractous lens: (Fig. 19 (A-Z))

Phacoemulsification was first introduced by Kelman in 1967(48). The procedure involves ultrasonic fragmentation and aspiration of the cataractous lens through a small incision. Phacoemulsification permit removal of a cataractous lens through a small incision, eliminate some of the complications associated with ECCE, and shorten the recovery period.

A clear corneal incision (main port) using a 2.8 mm angled keratome is given at about 1 mm anterior to the limbus. The anterior chamber is then filled with Trypan blue. Two minutes later the remaining dye is removed by washing the anterior chamber with lactated Ringer's. Later the anterior chamber volume is restored with viscoelastic agent (2% hydroxypropyl methyl cellulose). Continuous anterior capsulorrhexis capsulectomy is performed using an Utrata capsulorrhexis forceps, to remove a piece of anterior capsule (about 5-6 mm) to facilitate the entry of phaco-needle for endocapsular phacoemulsification of cataractous lens.

A second 1 mm corneal incision (side port) is made using a 15° lancet about 80-90° from the first incision to admit other instruments such as nuclear manipulator. In the next step, hydrodissection with the help of a 27 g cannula loaded onto a two ml syringe is performed by carefully injecting lactated Ringer's between the anterior lens capsule and the cortex to loosen the outer cortex from the lens capsule.

After anterior capsulectomy and hydrodissection, the phaco hand piece is carefully inserted through the main port corneal incision and capsulectomy site to sculpt the central portion of the cataractous lens, followed by nuclear rotation and phacoemulsification. The sculpting is initially limited to the nucleus, fragmenting it into small pieces, and then removing it. The remaining nucleus and cortices are fragmented by parallel sculpting. After fragmentation and aspiration of most of the cataractous lens material, any remaining material should be carefully removed, avoiding tearing of the posterior lens capsule. An irrigation–aspiration hand-piece is used to finally remove any remaining cataractous material from the equator and surface of the posterior lens capsule. The eye lids were closed by temporary tarsorrahphy suture using 2 – 0 silk thread. Phacoemulsification is the technique of choice for cataract extraction in dogs.

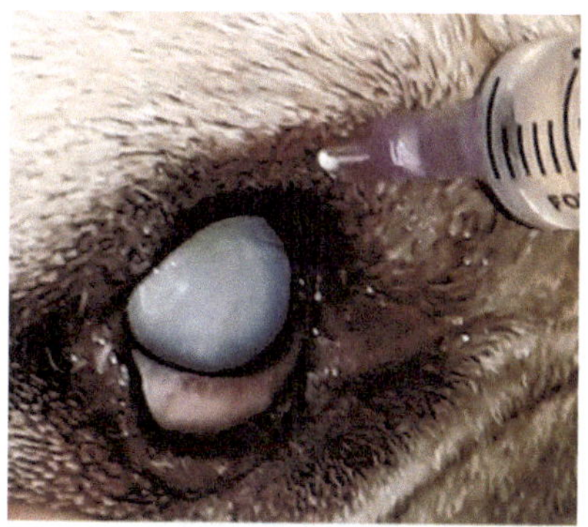

A. Retrobulbar injection of 2% lignocaine hcl.

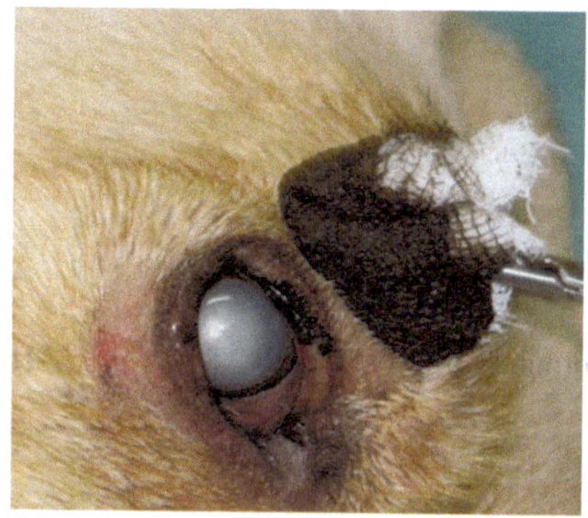

B. Painting of surrounding surgical site with povidone iodine

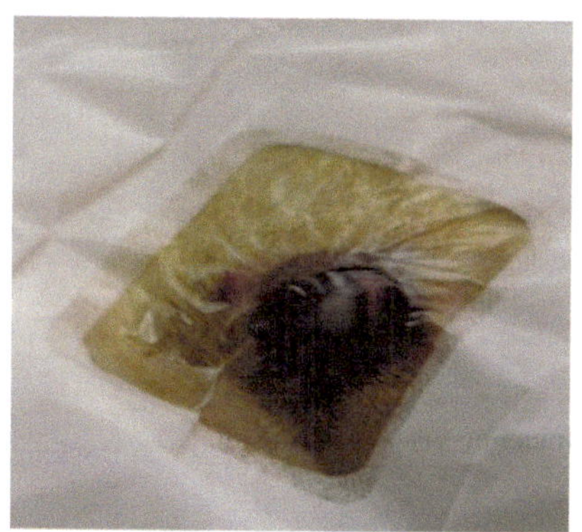

C. Draping of eye

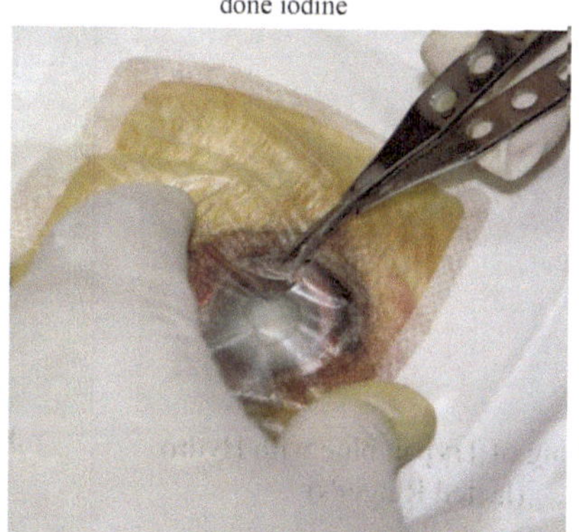

D. Drape window opening

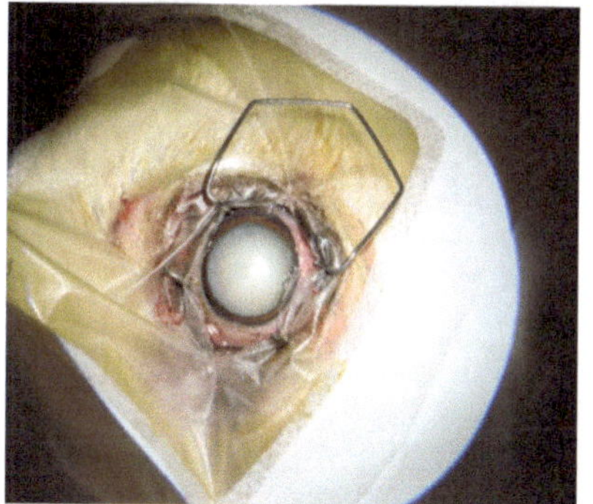

E. Application of eye speculum

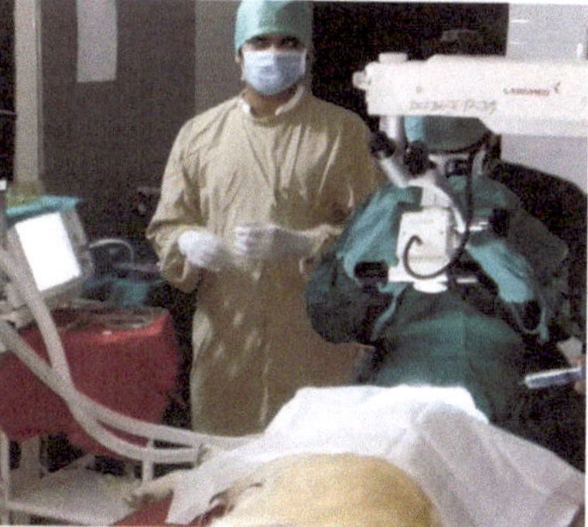

F. Final positioning under operating microscope

Operative Procedure

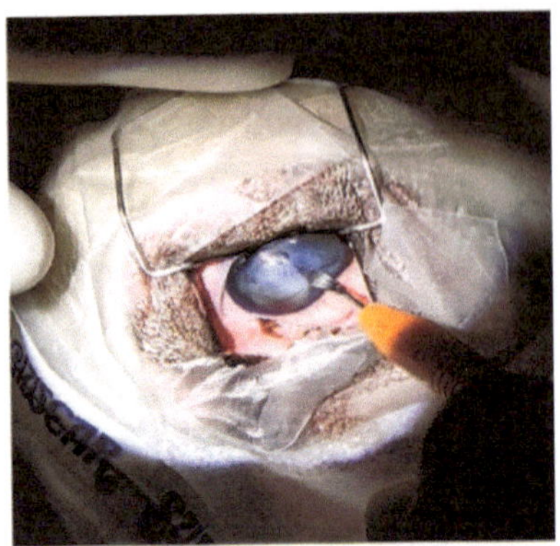

G. Performing corneal stab with 2.8 mm keratone

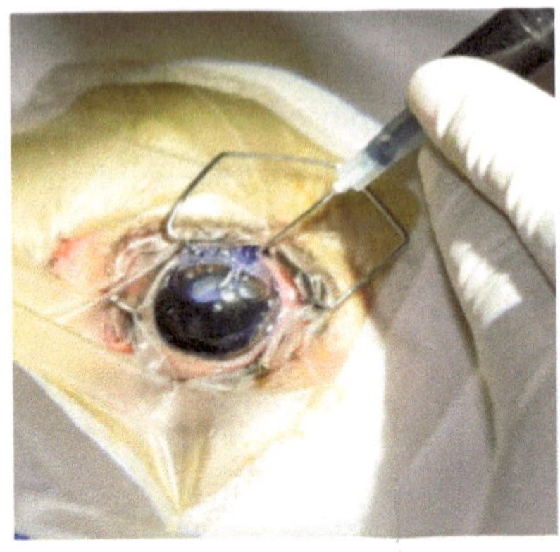

H. Anterior capsule staining with Trypan blue

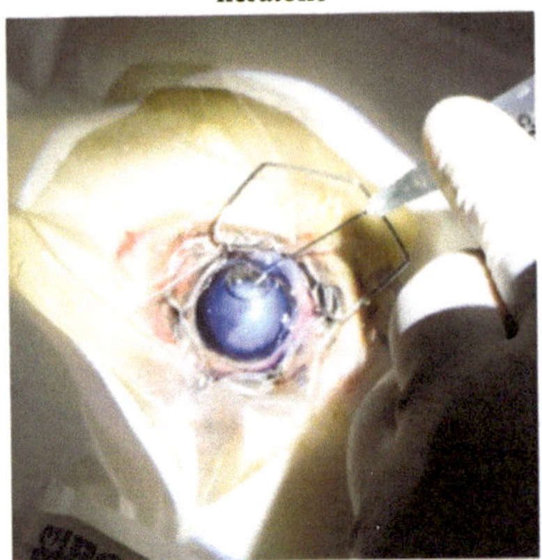

I. Flushing of Trypan blue with Hydro (lacted Ringer's)

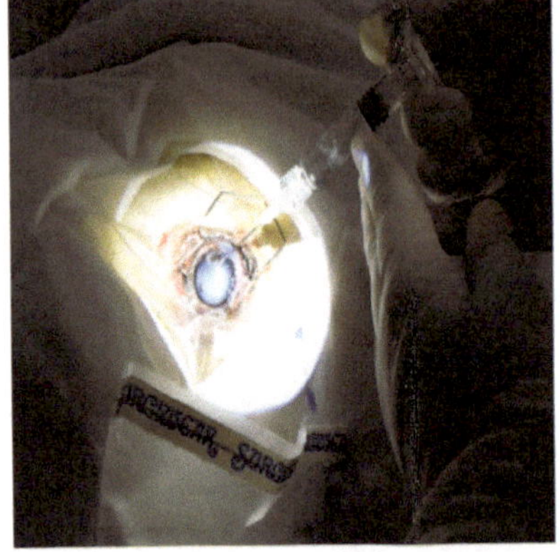

J. Injecting viscoelastic agent

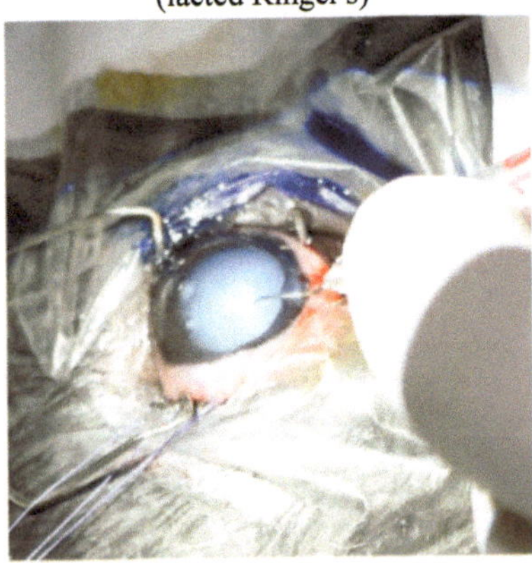

K. Giving a cut in anterior lens capsule with 26 gauge needle

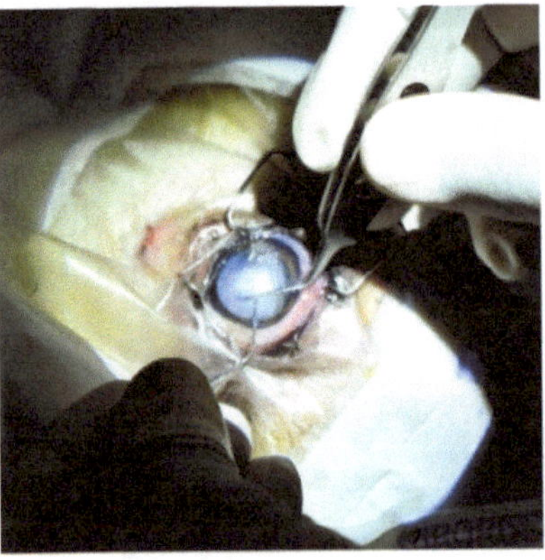

L. Capsulorrhexis using Utrata forceps

Operative Procedure

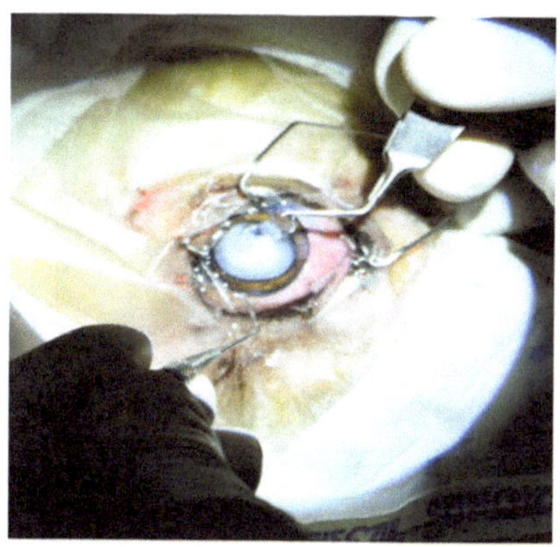

M. Capsulorrhexis complete and a piece of anterior lens capsule is removed

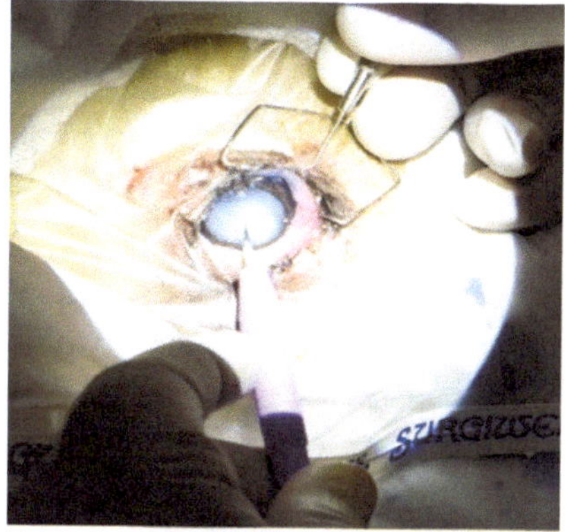

N. Creating side port entry with 15° lance tip blade

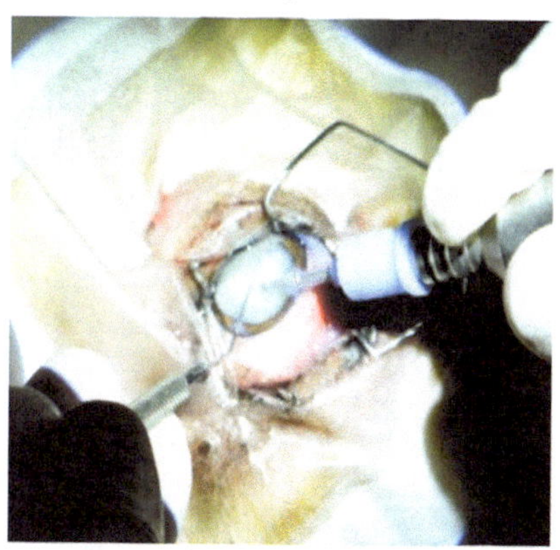

O. Creating Initial deep trench

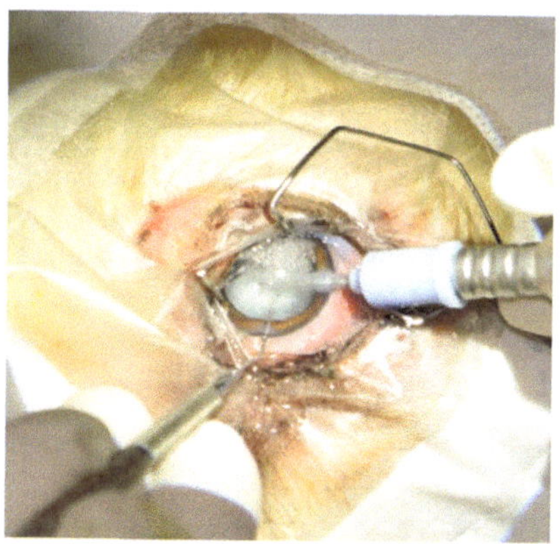

P. Sculpting

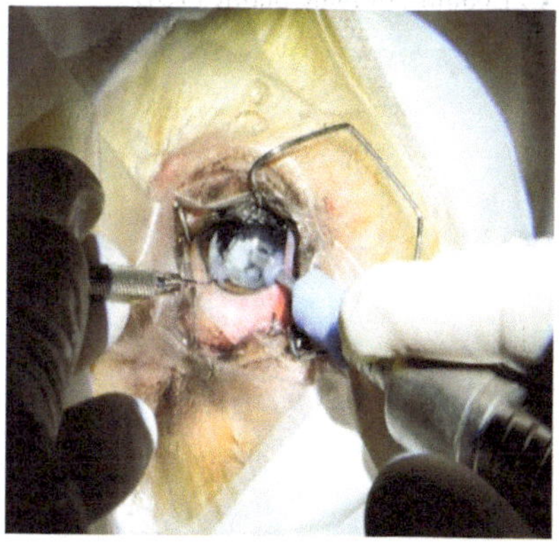

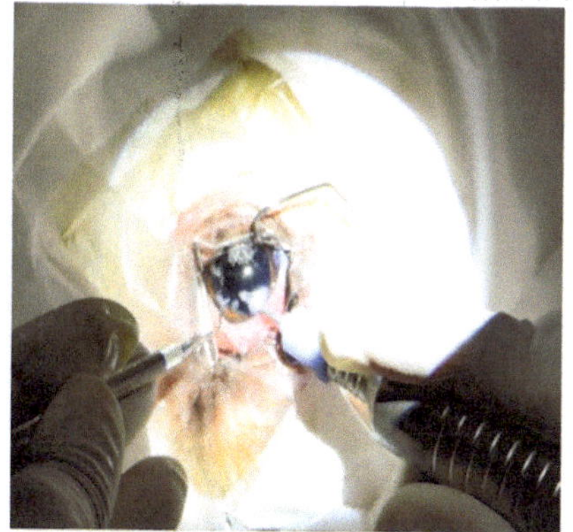

Q. Phaco-fragmentation and aspiration

Operative Procedure

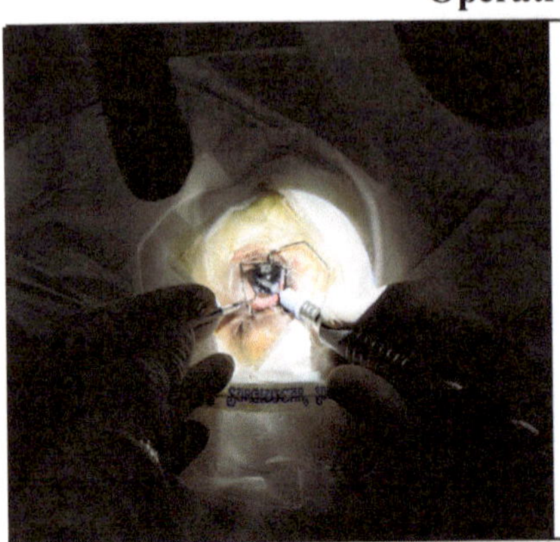

R. Final cortical clean up

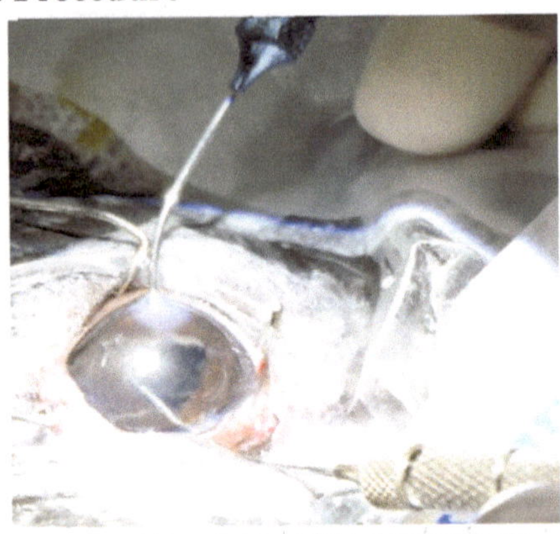

S. Final cleanup with irrigation aspiration unit

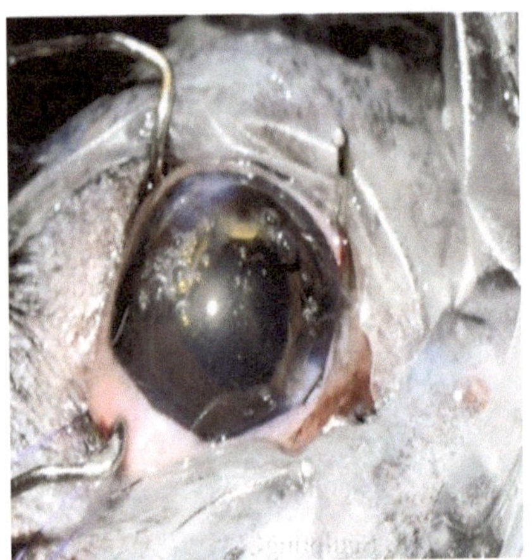

T. Immediate postoperative view of the eye

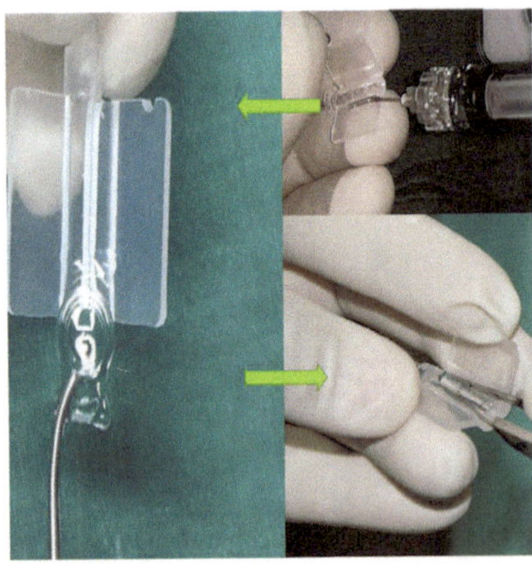

U. Loading of plate haptics IOL

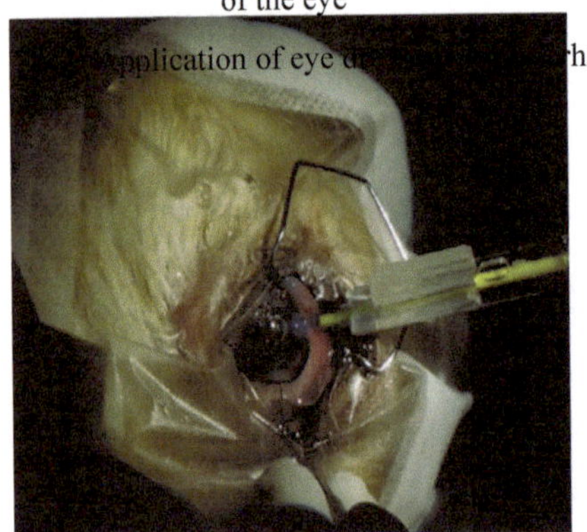

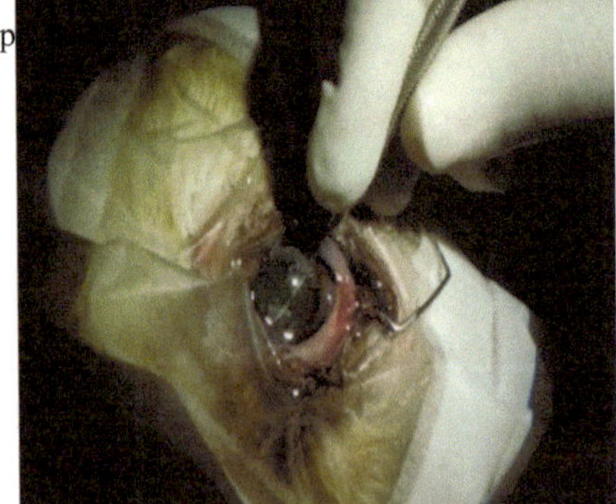

V&W. IOL implantation in the capsular bag

Operative Procedure

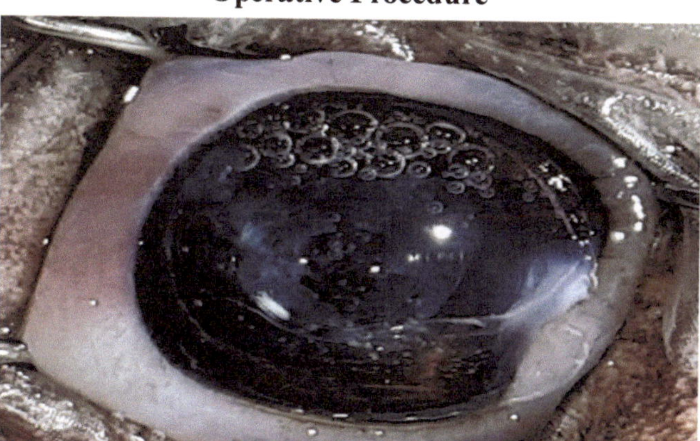

X. Immediate post operative view

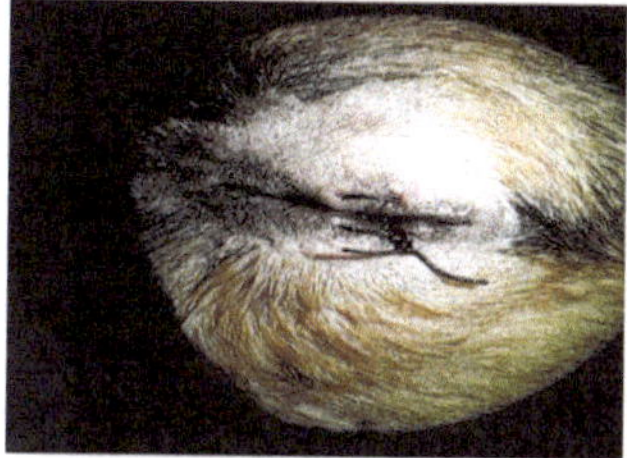

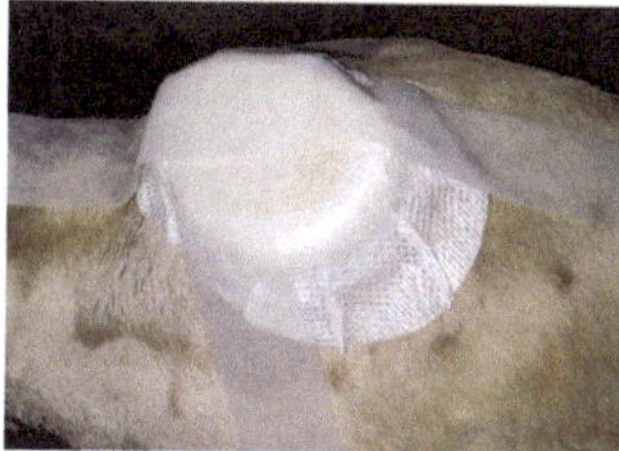

Y&Z. Application of eye dress after tarsorrhaphy satures

Fig. 19: Operative Procedure

Post-Operative Care (Fig. 20)

All the dogs are required to wear Elizabethan collar at all times during the first three weeks to prevent self-trauma. The owners are advised to avoid excitement or any compelling factors to dogs to minimize post-operative complications. Eye lid sutures are removed on the next days to surgery. The exterior of operated eye is cleaned daily with Luke warm distilled water for seven days. A broad-spectrum systemic antibiotic is given for 7 days. Tab. Acetazolamide 250 mg may be prescribed @ 10 mg/ kg orally, in two divided doses for 7 days to eliminate postoperative glaucoma. Mydriasis is maintained using atropine drops t.i.d for first three days to check uveitis.

Eye drops Difluprednate b.i.d for 1st week are instilled in cases where corneal opacity is suspected. Eye drops Moxifloxacin four times a day for 1st week, t.i.d. for 2nd week and b.i.d for next 15 days and eye drops Flurbiprofen are instilled for every hour a day for 15 days and. Medications and doses are changed based on intraocular complications. Thus the frequency of eye drops is tapered down and stopped after one month.

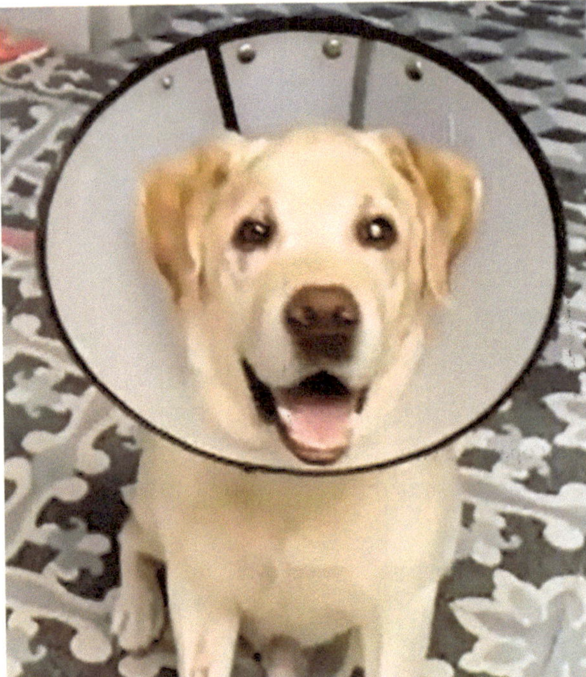

Dog wearing elizabethan collar

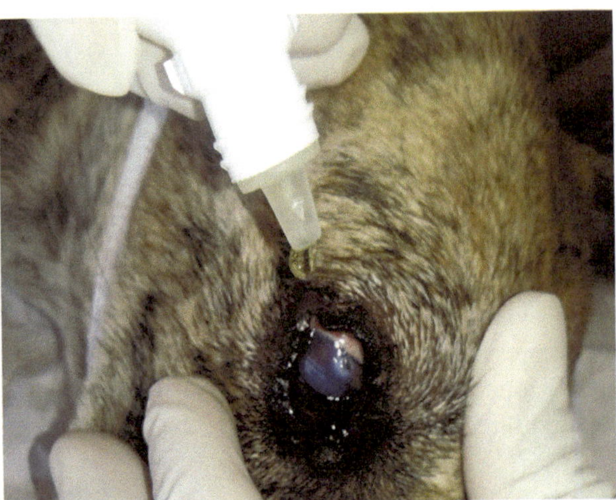

Instillation of eye drops

Fig. 20: Postoperative Care

6

Complications of Cataract Surgery

Intra-operative complications

Although the phacoemulsification technique costs higher, it provides shorter surgical time and less complication than extracapsular lens extraction (49).

The most important intraoperative complications are anterior capsular fibrosis, radial tear of anterior capsule, posterior capsular rupture, vitreous prolapse and post-operative complications like uveitis and corneal oedema (50).

The production of ultrasound energy in phacoemulsification is associated with heat generation that can result in damage to ocular tissue, in particular the corneo-scleral wound site. Thermal damage to the corneo-scleral wound site may result in difficulty with wound closure and consequent risk of wound leakage, as well as damage to the adjacent corneal stroma and endothelium, fistula formation, and the induction of high degrees of post-operative astigmatism. The loss of adequate flow of irrigation fluid around the phacoemulsification tip is the key factor in the development of phacoemulsification-induced thermal injury. Use of excessive ultrasound power and production of excessive frictional forces generated by contact of the vibrating phacoemulsification needle with the irrigation sleeve are also factors involved (51).

Besides these, intraoperative complication at different point of time during the surgery includes blood in the anterior chamber (hyphema) and pupil constriction (miosis) (52).

Post-operative complications

Phaco fragmentation is the most successful technique in the dog however; postoperative complications such as uveitis, hyphema, glaucoma, capsular opacities, corneal endothelial damage, and retinal detachment may be recorded following the surgery (53). However, suture dehiscence and iris prolapse are the common complications in case of ECCE.

The complications associated with polymethyl methacrylate intraocular lens implantation in canines include haptic dislocation, pupillary capture, pseudoaphakic corneal edema and pseudoaphakic precipitates, which may develop several years after cataract surgery (54).

Literature Cited

1. Gould, D. (2002). Clinical assessment of cataract in dogs. In Practice, 24: 28-34.
2. Dziezyc, J. (1990). .Cataract Surgery. Current approaches. Veterinary Clinics of North America: Small Animal Practice 20 (3): 737-754.
3. Gelatt, K.N. and Gelatt, J.P., (2001). Surgical procedures of the lens and cataracts. In: Gelatt KN, Gelatt JP (eds.). Small Animal Ophthalmic Surgery: Practical Techniques for the Veterinarian, Butterworth-Heinemann, Oxford, UK: 286-334.
4. Kecova, H. S. and Necas, A. (2004). Phacoemulsification and intraocular lens Implantation: Recent Trends in Catract Surgery. ACTA VET. BRNO: 73 85-92.
5. Ofri, R. (2013). Lens. In: MAGGS, D.J.; NILLER, P.E.; OFRI, R. (Eds.). Slatter's Fundamentals of Veterinary Ophthalmology. Gainesville: Elsevier .272- 290.
6. Ofri, R. (2008 b). Lens. In: Maggs D.J, Miller P.E. and Ofri, R. (Eds.). Slatter's Fundamentals of Veterinary Ophthalmology (4th ed.): 258-276. St. Louis: Saunders, USA.
7. Magrane, W. G. (1971). The Normal Eye: Canine Ophthalmology. 2nd ed., Lea and Febiger, Philadelphia, USA: 3-5.
8. Beteg, F., Mates, N. and Muste, A. (2006). Cataracts in dog And actually trends in opacified lens removal. Bulletin UASVM-CN, Veterinary Medicine 63: 186-198.
9. Collins, B.K., Collier, L. L., Johnson, G.S., Shibuya, H., Moore, C.P. and daSilva Curiel, J.M.A. (1992). Familial cataracts and concurrent ocular anomalies in Chow Chows. Journal of American Veterinary Medical Association. 200(10), May15:1485-1491.
10. Rose, M.D., Mattoon, J. S., Gemensky-Metzler, A. J., Wilkie, D.A., Rajala-Schultz, P.J. (2008). Ultrasound biomicroscopy of the iridocorneal angle of the eye before and after phacoemulsification and intraocular lens implantation in dogs. AJVR, 69(2): 279-288.
11. Williams, D.L., Heath, M.F. and Wallis, C. (2004). Prevalence of canine cataract: preliminary results of a cross sectional study. Veterinary Ophthalmology. 7(1). 29-35.
12. Ramani, C., Manjokumar, A., Shafiuzama, Md., Nitin, J. D. and Nagarajan, L. (2013). Incidence of cataract in dogs: A retrospective study. Tamilnadu J. Vet. Ani. Sci., 9 (3), 231-233.
13. Ofri, R. (2008 a). Cataracts: causes and Classification. Ophthalmology, Scientific Proceedings: Companion Animals Programme 1,: 171-172.
14. Elder, D. and Sir, S. (1969). System of Ophthalmology, Vol. XI, C. V. Mosby Co., St. Louis.
15. Gelatt, K.N. (1974). Traumatic cataract and optic nerve atrophy in a dog. Veterinary Medicine Small Animal Clinics 69: 988.
16. Van Heyningen (1976). Experimental studies on cataracts. Invest Ophthalmol. 15 : 685.
17. Andley, U. P. and Clark, B. A. (1989). Generation of oxidants in the near UV photo oxidation of human lens a crystalline. Invest. Ophthalmol. Vis. Sci., 30 (4), 706-713
18. Engle, R. and Spencer, W. (1995). Lens, in Spencer W (ed). Ophthalmic Pathology. Philadelphia, WB Saunders: 372-427.
19. Feldman, E.C. and Nelson, R.W. (2004). Canine diabetes mellitus, in Canine and Feline Endocrinology and Reproduction, ed 3. St. Louis, Saunders W.B.: 486–538.

20. Koch, S. A. and Rubin, L. F. (1967). Probable nonhereditary congenital cataract in dogs. J. Am. Vet. Med. Assoc. 150:1374.
21. Gelatt, K. N. (1972). Cataracts in the Golden Retriever dog. Vet. Med. Small. Anim. Clin. 67: 113.
22. Ori, J.I., Yoshikai, T., Yoshimur, S., Ujino, H. and Takase, K. (2000). Posterior lenticonus with congenital cataract in a Shih Tzu dog. The Journal of Veterinary Medical Science, 62, 1201–1203.
23. Rubin, L. F. and Flower, R. D. (1972). Inherited cataract in a family of Standard Poodle. J. Am. Vet. Med. Assoc. 161: 207.
24. Davidson, H.J and Keil, S.M (2001). Canine cataracts: A review of diagnostic and treatment procedure. Journal of Veterinary Medicine. 96: 14-38.
25. Barnett, K.C. (1978). Hereditary cataract in the dog. Journal of Small Animal Practice 19: 109-120.
26. Bagley, L.H. and Lavach, J.D. (1994). Comparison of postoperative phacoemulsification results in dogs with and without diabetes mellitus: 153 cases (1991-1992) Journal of the American Veterinary Medical Association 205, 1165-1169.
27. Peiffer, R. C., Gelatt, K. N. and Gwin, R. M. (1977). Diabetic cataract in the dogs. Can. Pract., 4, 18-22.
28. Kornegay, J., Greene, C., Martin, C., Gorgacz, E. and Melcon, D. (1980). Idiopathic hypocalcemia in four dogs. Journal of the American Animal Hospital Association 16: 723–734.
29. Paterson, C. and Delamere, N. (1992). The lens. Adler's Physiology of the Eye, 9th edn. W Hart (ed). Mosby Year Book, St Louis: 348–390.
30. Ashton, N., Brown, N. and Easty, D. (1969). Trematode cataract in fresh-water fish. Transactions of the Ophth. Soc. of the UK. 89: 263-278.
31. Sanford, S., Dukes, E. and Thomas, W. (1978). Acquired bilateral cortical cataracts in mature sows. J. Am. Vet. Med. Assoc., 173 (7), 852-853.
32. Martin, C.L., Christmas, R., and Leipold, H. (1972). Formation of temporary cataracts in dogs given a disophenol preparation. Journal of the American Veterinary Medical Association 161: 294–301.
33. Martin, C. L. (1975). The Formation of Cataracts in dogs with Disphenol: Age Susceptibility and Production with chemical grade 2, 6-diiodo-4-nitrophenol. Can.Vet.J. 16 : 228.
34. Gwin, R. M. and Gelatt, K. N. (1985). Ophthalmic Anatomy. In K. N. Gelatt (Ed.), Veterinary Ophthalmology (3rd ed., pp. 440-442) Lippincott, Williams and Wilkins, Philadelphia.
35. Gelatt, K. N. and Wilkie, D.A. (2011). Surgical procedures of the lens and cataracts. In: Veterinary Ophthalmic Surgery:, eds. Gellat, K. N. and Gellat, J.P., Elsevier Saunders, Gainesville, FL USA: 312-330.
36. Ofri, R. (2006). Ocular examination. Paper presented at the World Small Animal Veterinary Association World Congress. Retrieved from www.ivis.org/proceedings/wsava/2006/lecture21/Ofri3.pdf?LA=1
37. Gelatt, K.N. (2014). Eye examination and diagnostics. In Essentials of Veterinary Ophthalmology, 3rd ed., John Wiley and Sons.Inc: 103-144.
38. Moore, P. A. (2001). Examination technique and interpretation of ophthalmic findings. Clinical techniques in small animal practice. 16 (1), 1-12.
39. Adkins, A. E. and Hendrix, D.V.H. (2003). Cataract Evaluation and Treatment in Dog: A review. Compendium on Continuing Education for the Practicing Veterinarian, 25(11),812. Retrievedfromhttp://works.bepress.com/diane_hendrix/24/.

40. Maggs, D. J. (2013). Basic diagnostic techniques. In Maggs, D. J., Miller, P. and Ofri, R. (Eds.). Slatter's Fundamentals of Veterinary Ophthalmology (4th ed.): 79- 109, Saunders, Philadelphia.
41. Park, S.A., Yi, N.Y., Jeong, M.B., Kim, W.T, Kim, S.E., Chae, J.M. and Seo, K.M. (2009). Clinical manifestations of cataracts in small breed dogs. Veterinary Ophthalmology. 12, 4: 205–210.
42. Schmid, V (2006). Imaging of the Eye and Orbit: 278-300. In Diagnostic Ultrasound in Small Animal practice Ed. Mannion, P, Blackwell Science Ltd, a Blackwell Publishing company, 9600 Garsington Road, Oxford OX4 2DQ, UK.
43. Martin, C. L. (2010). Lens. In: Opthalmic Disease in Veterinary Medicine (369-395). Manson Publishing Ltd., London, UK.
44. Narfstrom, K., Ekesten, B., Rosolen, S. G., Spiess, B. M., Percicot, C. L. and Ofri, R. (2002). Guideline for clinical electroretinography in the dog. Doc Ophthalmol. 105: 83-92.
45. Plummer, C. E., Specht, A. and Gelatt, K. N. (2007). Ocular manifestations of endocrine disease. Compendium, 2, 733-743.
46. Burwell, R. (2004). Assessing a patient for Cataract Surgery, Ocular Outlook 3(5): 1- 3.
47. Moore, C.P. (1999). Diseases and surgery of the lacrimal secretory system, in Gelatt KN (ed). Veterinary Ophthalmology, ed.3. Philadelphia, Lippincott Williams and Wilkins, pp 583–607.
48. Kelman, C.D. (1994). The history and development of phacoemulsification. Int Ophthalmol Clin 34: 1-12.
49. Laus, J. L., Pigatto, A. T., Jorge, A. T., Oria, P. A., Santos, C. and Rezende, M. L.(2002). Phacoemulsification Versus Extra Capsular Lens Extraction in dogs. (Paper published in 27th World Congress of WSAVA).
50. Zgencül, F. E. (2005). The results of phacofragmentation and aspiration surgery for cataract extraction in dogs. Turk. J. Vet. Anim. Sci. 29: 165-173.
51. Sippel, K.C.andPineda, R. Jr.(2002). Phacoemulsification and thermal wound injury. Semin Ophthalmol. Sep-Dec; 17(3-4), 102-9.
52. Ahmad, R., Saini, N.S., Mahajan, S.K., Mohindroo, J. and Singh, S.S. (2017). Comparison of rigid polymethylmethacrylate and foldable square edgeacrylic lens replacement for management of cataract after phacoemulsification in 22 eyes of dogs.Indian J. Anim. Res., 51 (1) 2017: 146-150.
53. Whitley, R. D., McLaghlin, S. A., Whitley, E. M. and Gilger, B. C. (1993). Cataract removal in dogs: The surgical techniques. Vet. Med. 12 (9): 859-66.
54. Gaiddon, J.A., Lallement, P.E., Jr, R.L.P. (2000).Implantation of a foldable intraocular lens in dogs. Journal of American Veterinary Medical Association. 216(6): 875-877.

Subject Index

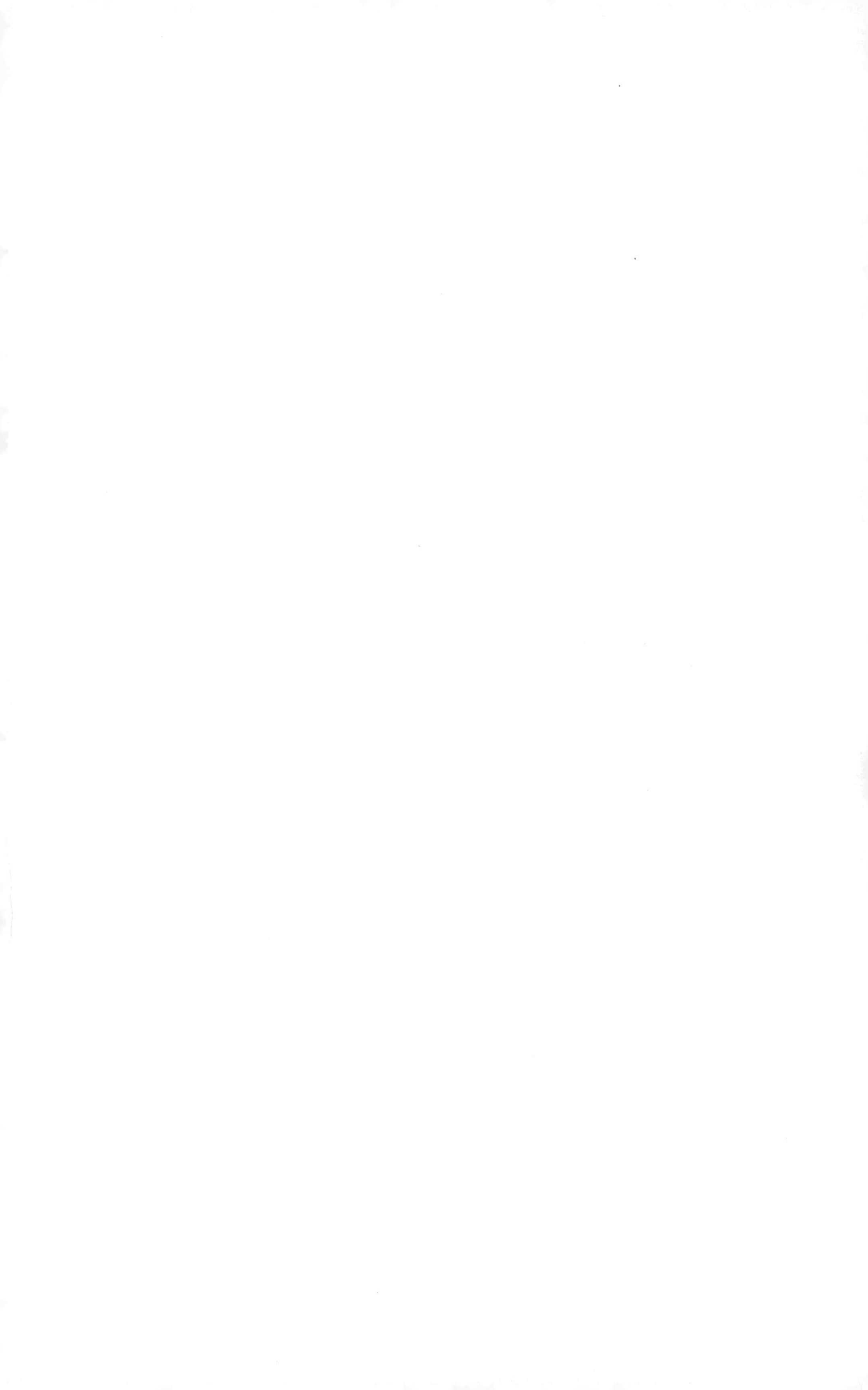

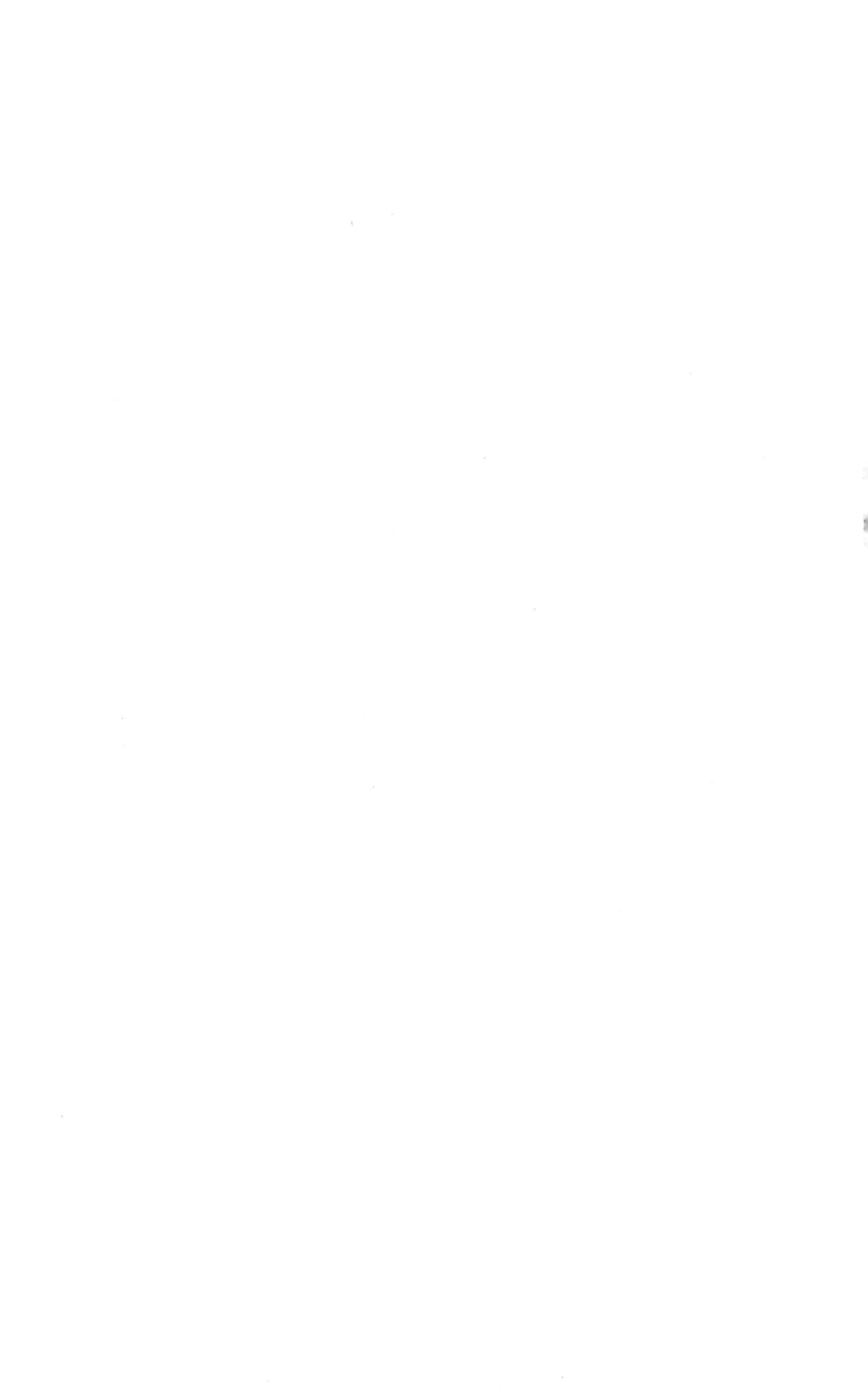